Kriya Yoga Sūtras of Patañjali and the Siddhas

Translation, Commentary, and Practice
By M. Govindan

Kriya Yoga Publications

St. Etienne de Bolton, Quebec, Canada

Kriya Yoga Sūtras of Patañjali and the Siddhas

Translation, Commentary and Practice
By M. Govindan

First published in December 2000
Second published in November 2005 by
Kriya Yoga Publications
196 Mountain Road, P.O. Box 90
Eastman, Quebec, Canada J0E 1P0
Telephone: 450-297-0258; 1-888-252-9642; fax: 450-297-3957
www.babaji.ca email: info@babaji.ca

Cover design: Uwe Haardt, Circular painting of Patañjali on the front cover and Tirumūlar on the rear cover are from the ceiling of the Chidambaram Temple. The painting of the 18 Siddhas on the rear cover is from the Saraswati Mahal Museum in Tanjore, Tamil Nadu, India

Printed and bound in Canada.

Canadian Cataloguing in Publication Data
Govindan, Marshall
Kriya yoga sūtras of Patañjali and the Siddhas

Includes bibliographical references and index
ISBN 1-895383-12-9

1. Patañjali. Yoga sūtra. 2. Yoga-Early works to 1800. 3. Yoga, Kriya. I. Govindan, Marshall II. Title.

B132.Y6P27 2000 181'.452C00-901057-2

Dedicated to
Babaji Nagaraj,
Patañjali
&
all other members of the
18 Siddha Kriya Yoga Tradition

Table of Contents

Acknowledgements

The author is very grateful to everyone who supported him in preparing this work. In particular, I would like to thank:

- Durga Ahlund for many of the "practices" suggested in the commentary, many of the commentaries themselves, as well as for her assistance in finding many of the quotations from Sri Aurobindo and the Mother. Also, in the laborious task of preparing the Index of Sanskrit Words and the Index of English Words in the Sutras.

- Sujata Ghosh, for her review and correction of the Sanskrit translation and many thoughtful suggestions regarding the commentary.

- Maureen Mueller for her editing and many helpful comments, suggestions, and overall encouragement.

- Uwe Haardt for the design of cover and rear cover pages.

- Georg Feuerstein, for reviewing this manuscript and for some very helpful suggestions. I would also like to acknowledge how grateful I am to him for his great scholarship in preparing my principal reference, his book "Yoga-Sutras: A New Translation and Commentary.

- Bob Butera, for his comments and suggestions regarding the manuscript, which helped me to make it more complete and useful.

- Jay Ganesha Valinsky for the formatting of the final text.

- To the many students with whom I shared these commentaries over the past ten years: for their feedback on the commentaries, as well as for their financial support in bringing out this publication.

• Yogi Ramaiah, who first introduced me to Patanjali and taught me the method of how to meditate upon his Sutras, as well as the 144 Kriyas in Babaji's Kriya Yoga.

• Babaji Nagaraj for guiding me in the preparation of this work and for bringing to his disciples the wonderful system of 144 Kriyas in his Kriya Yoga, referred to throughout this commentary. Whatever inspiration has come to me is due to His grace.

• Siddha Patañjali, whose masterful work has inspired me for more than 30 years.

• All of the Yoga Siddhas, for having developed Kriya Yoga. Their example inspires me daily.

• To all of them, I offer my heartfelt thanks. May all of you, dear readers, become Self-realized through their labor of love.

Marshall Govindan
www.babaji.ca

December 7, 2000

Notes to Translation

Much care has been take to ensure that this translation reflects faithfully and literally the original Sanskrit. However, in some verses, where a literal translation left the meaning too obscure, a freer, more interpretive translation has been allowed. In balancing the need for precision with that of comprehension, this translation favors precision. A more complete understanding may be obtained by studying the word by word translation for each verse, which contains alternative meanings for the Sanskrit, as indicated in standard references and other recognized translations of this work. The commentary itself will also serve to fill in any gaps in comprehension of the translation.

All words appearing in parentheses are in the Sanskrit language, unless otherwise indicated. For example (Tam.) indicates the word is of Tamil origin.

Guide to the Pronunciation of Sanskrit

a	c*u*t
ā	f*a*ther
i	l*i*ly
ī	f*ee*t
u	c*ou*p
ū	b*oo*
ṛ	p*r*etty
ṝ	ma*r*ine
ḷ	reve*lr*y
ḹ	reve*lr*y (long)
e	grey
ai	*e*ye
o	r*o*pe
au	s*ou*nd
k	*c*ut
kh	in*kh*orn
g	*g*ate
gh	fo*gh*orn
ṅ	si*ng*
c	*ch*ase
ch	chur*ch*ill
j	*j*et
jh	hed*geh*og
ñ	stra*n*ge (nasal)
ṭ	*t*rue
ṭh	an*th*ill
ḍ	*d*rum
ḍh	mu*dh*ut
ṇ	*n*avel
t	*t*ake
th	nu*th*ook (dental)
d	*d*ate
dh	a*dh*ere
n	*n*ot
p	cli*p*
ph	u*ph*ill
b	tu*b*
bh	a*bh*or
m	ri*m*
y	ro*y*al
r	*r*ed
l	*l*ane
v	*v*anish
ś	*s*ure
ṣ	bu*sh*
s	*s*aint
h	*h*appiness

Foreword

by Georg Feuerstein, Ph.D.

Today tens of millions of people around the world practice *Yoga* of one kind or another. Often what they practice barely resembles traditional *Yoga*, as it has been pursued over five millennia in India. Therefore there is a real need for sincere voices like that of Marshall Govindan, who stands for authentic *Yoga*, which is always concerned with the great ideal of profound personal transformation and liberation. Govindan, as he prefers to be called, represents the tradition of *Kriya Yoga (Skt.kriyā yoga)*, which was first taught by the Himālayan adept known as Babaji and has been handed down through several teaching lineages. Govindan was initiated into *Kriya Yoga* by Yogi S. A. A. Ramaiah and since 1988 has himself initiated thousands of students.

S. A. A. Ramaiah is a South Indian master who claims to have been initiated directly by Babaji, best known from Paramahaṁsa Yogānanda's *Autobiography of a Yogi*, as one of the immortal adepts of *Siddha Yoga*. According to Govindan's *Babaji and the 18 Siddha Kriya Yoga Tradition*, Yogi Ramaiah has provided some biographical details about that great adept, including his birthdate of November 30, 203 AD Apparently, Babaji was a disciple of *Pōkanāthar (Tam.* pronounced Boganathar), who presided over the temple of *Katirgama* (Skt. *Karttikeyagrāma*) to be found in a forest at the southernmost tip of Sri Lanka. At a certain point, *Pōkanāthar* sent his disciple to the great adept Agastyar under whose guidance Babaji achieved liberation and immortality.

Another great master of South Indian Siddha Yoga was Tirumūlar, the author of the well-known Tamil *Tirumantiram* (*Tam.* pronounced *Tirumandiram).* In this work, Tirumūlar speaks of himself as a disciple of Naṇḍi, who apparently also taught a certain Patañjali. Few Western students of *Yoga* have heard of Tirumūlar, but they know Patañjali, the compiler of the famous *Yoga-Sūtras.* This aphoristic work masterfully maps out the *yogic* path from a philosophical and psychological perspective.

The *Yoga-Sūtras* are generally assigned to the period between 200 BC and 200 AD. The former date is generally favored by those who identify the compiler of the *Sūtras* with the famous grammarian Patañjali. More and more scholars, however, opt for the latter date, which takes into account that the *Yoga-Sūtras* reflect the language and conceptual universe of Mahāyāṇa Buddhism.

Tradition knows of several other individuals by the name of Patañjali, including the *Sāṁkhya* authority and a composer of a *Sūtric* work on ritual. Virtually nothing is known about them or their dates. Tirumūlar's mention of a fellow disciple called Patañjali further muddies the historical waters.

Most scholars place Tirumūlar between the first and seventh century AD. The ideas and practices found in the *Tirumantiram*, however, represent a stage of development of Hindu *Tantra* that suggests a date between the fifth and tenth century AD. If correct, this would make Tirumūlar's fellow disciple Patañjali someone other than the compiler of the *Yoga-Sutra*. But regardless of such scholarly considerations, a comparison between the *Yoga-Sūtras* and the *Tirumantiram* is important and long overdue.

For the past 35 years, my research into *Yoga* has been focused on the Sanskrit sources. I first encountered the *Tirumantiram*, which is written in Tamil, in 1998 in the edition arranged and published by Govindan five years earlier. I had of course known of the *Tirumantiram* many years earlier, having myself republished in 1993 *The Poets of the Powers* by the renowned scholar of Tamil Kamil V. Zvelebil, who described Tirumūlar as "the foremost exponent of Yoga in Tamil" (p. 38). Zvelebil's short quotations from Tirumular's work intrigued me greatly, and thus B. Natarajan's English rendering of the *Tirumantiram*, published by Govindan, was an incredible find for me. I readily appreciated the enormous depth of Tirumūlar's treatment of *Yoga* and in the meantime have come to believe that all students of *Yoga* should carefully study the *Tirumantiram* alongside the *Yoga-Sūtras* and the *Bhagavad-Gīta*.

The present book examines Patañjali's *Yoga-Sūtras* in the light of the *Siddha Yoga* of Tamilnadu. Govindan has spared no effort to make the aphorisms accessible to those interested in yogic *practice*. In particular, the growing number of students of *Kriya Yoga* throughout the world will find his treatment indispensable, but others too will benefit from it.

It is most curious that while Patañjali's teaching has become virtually equated with eight-limbed *Yoga (aṣṭāṅga-yoga)*, he himself called his path that of action Yoga *(kriyā-yoga)* in *pāda* 2.1. As I tried to show in my monograph *The Yoga-Sutra: An Exercise in the Methodology of Textual Analysis*, the aphorisms in the *Yoga-Sūtras* dealing specifically with the eight limbs appear to have been quoted by Patañjali or subsequently added to his text. There is no real satisfactory explanation for why Patañjali used the label *kriyā-yoga* for his teachings. However, if we assume with Govindan that the compiler of the *Yoga-Sūtras* was a fellow disciple of Tirumūlar, we have a direct link to the Tantric heritage of South India, which knows the term *kriyā-yoga* in the sense of ritual activity.

Study (*svadhyāya*) has always been an integral aspect of *Yoga*. Western students, in my opinion, need to take this yogic practice more seriously. Because of its succinctness and focus on essentials, the *Yoga-Sūtras* are ideally suited for in-depth study. Its approach is rational, systematic, and philosophical. In contrast, the *Tirumantiram* is ecstatic and poetic and filled with precious nuggets of yogic experience and wisdom. Both texts complement each other beautifully, and their combined study will be found illuminating and elevating. Govindan's book provides an excellent platform for such a study. He writes from his own long experience of *Kriya Yoga* and a deep love and respect for the heritage of *Yoga*.

I have known Govindan only for a couple of years but have become impressed with his sincerity as a *Yoga* practitioner and teacher. He is indefatigable in his commitment to the teachings of his *guru*, Babaji, and his many students around the world. His energy, modesty, and kindness are a clear indication of the efficacy of the teachings he is embodying and passing on to others.

Marshall Govindan's *Kriya Yoga Sūtras of Patañjali* is a valuable addition to the study of *Yoga* in general and the *Yoga-Sūtras* in particular. I can wholeheartedly recommend it.

Georg Feuerstein, Ph.D.
Yoga Research and Education Center
www.yrec.org Sept. 9, 2000

Introduction

A COMPARISON BETWEEN THE *YOGA-SŪTRAS* AND *TIRUMANTIRAM*

Many translations and commentaries have been made regarding Patañjali's *Yoga-Sūtras*. However, scholars have ignored the many similarities between the *Yoga-Sūtras* and the most important work on Yoga written by a Tamil Yoga Siddha, the "*Tirumandiram*" by Siddha Tirumūlar.**(1)** Both works are among the oldest to deal primarily with Yoga. Both works share many philosophical similarities, as summarized in the table below. Both works deal extensively with the "siddhis," or yogic miraculous powers. Both works describe practical methods of Yoga, leaving out many important details, as Siddha yogis generally do in their writings. The Siddhas left the most important details for initiation in person with their students or disciples. Both authors figure prominently among most lists of "the 18 Tamil Yoga Siddhas.**(2)**

There are some indications that Patañjali and Tirumūlar were contemporaries in south India, with its unique cultural outlook. While the dating of both works is difficult, most scholars fix Patañjali's "*Yoga-Sūtras*" around the 2nd to the 4th centuries A.D. and "*Tirumandiram*" around the 4th century to 5th century A.D. However, Tirumūlar claims that it required 3,000 years for him to write "*Tirumandiram*," and he also mentions that he and Patañjali had a common guru, Nandi. He also celebrates the visit of Patañjali to Chidambaram, where he himself resided. There are many indications that Patañjali, as well as Tirumūlar, were both prominent Siddhas, and shared much the same outlook. Understanding the ramifications of this will help all practitioners of Yoga to appreciate the objectives, philosophy and practice of Yoga.

The failure of scholars to notice the many common philosophical and theological doctrines common to both works may be due the fact that the *Yoga-Sūtras* were written in *Sanskrit* only, and the *Tirumandiram* in Tamil only. Neither has been translated into the other language. Most scholars tend to work only in one of these two. The Tamil literature in general, and the Tamil Siddhas literature in particular, has been mostly ignored by modern scholars. An English translation of the "*Tirumandiram*" has only been available since 1991, and consequently, few in the west have been equipped to make the comparison.

However, after many years of preparation, a major research project, "The Tamil Yoga Siddha Manuscript Project" is being launched, under the sponsorship of Babaji's Kriya Yoga Order of Acharyas, and the Yoga Research and Education Center (founded by Georg Feuerstein) to preserve, protect and evaluate for possible translation and publication several thousand manuscripts lying in various manuscript libraries of south India. The present work must therefore be considered only a preliminary, if not tentative effort to fill a huge hole in our understanding of the origins of Yoga. As the results of the above mentioned project are gradually developed, there will undoubtedly be revisions.

The present translation and commentary of the "*Yoga-Sūtras*" will serve to reveal and clarify to English readers many arcane subjects in both Classical Yoga and the philosophy of the Tamil Yoga Siddhas, known as Saiva Siddhantha, in the light of these two great seminal masterpieces. The premise of this commentary is that by comparing the two, a deeper understanding of each may be gained.

Previous translations have, in my opinion, either been so literal that their meaning could only be grasped with great difficulty, or so highly interpreted that the real meaning was largely lost. Due to the highly technical nature of the subject matter, and the general unfamiliarity of the average reader with the material, most translations have greatly diluted the rich meaning of the verses. This new translation seeks a middle ground between readability and meaningfulness. In developing this new translation and commentary, I am indebted to the authors of three previous translations in particular: those of G. Feuerstein**(3)**, Swami Satchitananda**(4)** and Swami Hariharananda Aranya**(5)**.

This translation and commentary has been developed over the past decade in order to serve the needs of initiates of Babaji's Kriya Yoga, whose lineage of Nandi, Agastyar, Boganathar and Babaji is a branch of the 18 Tamil Yoga Siddha lineage. Initiates are taught how to meditate on the verses of the Siddhas like Patañjali and Tirumūlar. Until now they have had to rely upon translations which were not well suited to their needs.

Much of the material in this new translation, particularly the material in the first "Pada" or book, has already been shared with them, during meditation group meetings organized by myself all over the world. Babaji's Kriya Yoga is a practical crystallization of the philosophic system known as "Saiva Siddhantha", which in turn is a synthesis of the teachings of the 18 Tamil Yoga Siddha tradition, of whom both Tirumūlar and Patañjali are celebrated members. In many of the commentaries I have referred to specific practices in Babaji's Kriya Yoga in order help the students of this tradition to better appreciate their importance of their practice. This translation and commentary, therefore, can be appreciated by any interested reader but more especially by initiates of Babaji's Kriya Yoga, who themselves have experienced much of what Patañjali is referring to.

I am indebted to Babaji for having handed down the method of meditating on the verses to capture their hidden meaning. Each verse is like a key. A key is a useless piece of metal, unless one knows how to insert it into a lock and how to turn it. Then, the key, or verse, if meditated upon, permits one to enter into a new space, where the esoteric, or hidden, meaning may be revealed. If not meditated upon, it may only remain as useless ink on paper. The Siddhas typically would meditate for up to a year before composing a single verse. That verse would be only a key or introduction to a greater, hidden meaning. The Siddhas often concealed the meaning of their verses in order to reserve their esoteric teachings only for those initiates who were sufficiently advanced to grasp their significance based upon prior experience. More details on the pan-Indian Siddha tradition may be found in the work of David Gordon White**(6)** and on the Tamil Yoga Siddhas in the work of Zvelebil**(7)** and Govindan.**(8)**

The following table will summarize many important similarities between these two works:

Yoga-Sūtras	***Tirumandiram***
Purusha (Self) and *Prakriti* (Nature) are both real	*Purusa* and *Prakriti* are both real
Ishvara is the special Self, Being the teacher of teachers	*Isha* or *Siva* is the Supreme Being
Dualistic - theistic *Samkhya*	Dualistic - Advaita: the one has become many; Agamas and Vedas

Yoga-Sūtras	Tirumandiram
Purusha is multiple, unlike Vedanta's singular Atman	Jiva (Pasu) is multiple and is becoming Siva; 3 fold classification
Ashtanga Yoga is a preliminary practice	Ashtanga Yoga is elaborated upon
Ishvara is Patañjali's teacher, and he is very devoted to Him	Nandi (Siva) is his guru; very devoted Him
Emphasizes need for surrender to the Lord	Emphasizes need for surrender to the Lord
Five afflictions	Five fetters, similar to *Yoga-Sūtras* affliction
Evolution in creation is real, and follows 24 "*tattvas*" or principles	Evolution in creation is real and follows 24 "*tattvas*" or follows 36, even 96 "tattvas"
Doctrine of karmas and transmigration	Same
Ethics of social equality	Same
Triple realities: Ishvara, Purusha, Prakriti	Same
3 sources of knowledge	Similar
Method: Kriya Yoga: detachment, intense practice and self study	Method: Kundalini yoga, including pranayama, mantras, yantras
Parinama: transformation is emphasized: a process of purification of afflictions	Similar; purification of stains
Samadhi or cognitive absorption is:	Analogous:
a) with or without a physical form as a basis	a) "being in proximity to the Lord"
b) with or without a subtle form as a basis	b) "being the Lord's friend"
c) with or without a "seed" remaining	c) "being one with the Lord"
Speaks of 68 "siddhis" or powers, including perfection of the body	Speaks of 65 "siddhis" or powers, including physical immortality
Scope is limited to yoga, philosophy, some social ethics	Scope is much broader, and includes yoga, philosophy, tantra, social ethics

This comparison is by no means exhaustive. The subject matter is vast. In attempting to create a synthesis, and to compare the two, I have sought to stimulate the reader to go beyond what is here. I would welcome any comments or suggestions for future editions.

There are important differences between the two works, including the following:

Yoga-Sūtras	***Tirumandiram***
Written in third person, in a dry formulistic style	Written in the first person, with great feeling
Written in Sanskrit	Written in Tamil, the language of the people regardless of caste or status
195 aphorisms	3,047 verses

The similarities far outweigh the differences. Far greater philosophical differences can be found between the Vedantic literature versus the *Yoga-Sūtras* and *Tirumandiram.*

In bringing out this work, I have wanted to stimulate, above all, a greater appreciation and understanding of Yoga, both in the west and in India. Today, there is in general, widespread ignorance of the fact that Yoga is not merely a form of physical exercise, however healthful and therapeutic, but that it offers to 21st century humanity solutions to some of our most important social problems as well as those in the realms of philosophy, psychology, theology, and even ecology. It aims at nothing less than the full blossoming of each and every human's potential as a perfected divine being: physically, vitally, mentally, intellectually and spiritually. Today, the world is faced with unprecedented challenges in the realms of social conflict, ecological destruction, economic distribution and growth, as well as health. The globalisation of a materialistic culture cannot solve problems which transcend material values. Only a widespread social movement, which will enable individuals to go beyond limited egoistic preoccupations, can ensure our continued survival and the resolution of these many complex problems.

I humbly suggest to you, the reader, that a profound understanding of these two works will permit you to become a part of the solution, rather than a part of the problem that ails society and this planet today. In studying them, I challenge the reader to question their own values, habits and motivations, and where needed, make radical changes. In the words of Sri Aurobindo, "what is needed is a revolution against human nature". The *Yoga-Sūtras* and *Tirumandiram* will provide us with the vision and understanding as to how to fulfil our potential. They are like a roadmap which indicates various destinations, as well as the obstacles and how to overcome them. The Kriya Yoga of Babaji and the Siddhas is like a powerful automobile, which can transport us great distances. Its practice requires diligent and continuous effort on our part. No intellectual understanding is sufficient for becoming enlightened! But the practice of Yoga without understanding is also very incomplete, and today this is what we find so widespread in contemporary schools of Yoga. Both the kriyas and the written teachings have their place in an integrated process. Without understanding of where we are going, it is like having an automobile, but no road map. In these two works we have a roadmap which is universal.

PATAÑJALI'S KRIYA YOGA: CONSTANT PRACTICE AND DETACHMENT

"*Abhyasa*" and "*Vairagya*"

Currently, there are a great many modern adaptations of Yoga, particularly in the Western countries, which are given without reference to the classic teachings. As with a tree which has been cut off from its roots, there is a great danger that one's practice of Yoga will not be sustained unless one continues to seek inspiration from its origins. The values which such teachings provide are a potent cultural antidote to the numbing values of 21st century materialism, which is too often concerned with technology and quick results, inside or outside the context of Yoga. Classical Yoga, as expounded by the Siddha Patañjali around the second century A.D., describes a path to Self-Realization in the second chapter or "*Pāda*" of his famous "*Yoga-Sūtras*". As we will see, it is even more important today than it was 2000 years ago.

Patañjali calls it "Kriya Yoga" in verse II.1: "*tapas svādhyāya-īśvara-praṇidhānā kriyā-yogaḥ.*" "Intense practice, self-study and devotion to the Lord constitute *kriyā yoga.*" In the first chapter verses I.12 to 16 "constant practice" (*abhyāsa*) and "detachment" (*vairāgya*) are prescribed as the means of Yoga. As few persons are naturally endowed with much inclination towards "abhyasa" and "vairagya", Patañjali prescribes preliminary practices in the second chapter. Feuerstein**(1)** has pointed out, however, that Patañjali's Yoga was not the "ashtanga" or "eight-limbed" Yoga, described in verses II.28 to III.8, as has been commonly thought by most translators. Textual analysis has revealed that these verses were merely quoted from another unknown source.**(2)** We will discuss first of all the relationship between these means and components of Patañjali's Kriya Yoga.

Feuerstein**(3)** has created the following tree diagram on the following page which shows the relationship between the two branches of his Kriya Yoga:

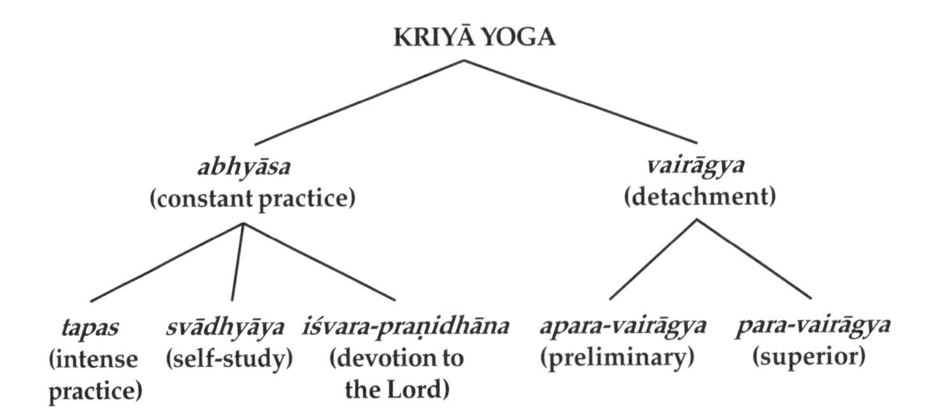

This vividly portrays the constant relationship between the two principal means of Kriya Yoga, "practice" and "detachment", as well as the essential components of practice, and the preliminary and superior forms of detachment.

In verse I.12 Patañjali says: "*abhyāsa-vairāgyābhyāṁ tan-nirodhaḥ*," "By constant practice and with detachment (arises) the cessation (of identifying with the fluctuations of consciousness)". By "constant practice" he refers to concentrating on what one truly is, the Self, or in preparatory exercises, on objects of concentration (as it is easier to concentrate on an object with form than on the formless Absolute). "Detachment" refers to letting go of or releasing what one is not: passing thoughts, emotions, sensations coming from the five sense organs. "Practice" and "detachment" can be thought of the as the two magnetic poles of any yogic discipline. The former represents the endeavour to actualize the Self by means of the techniques of interiorisation and experience of unity; the latter represents the corresponding attitude of "letting go" of the hunger for the external world of diversity.

"*Abhyasa*" (Practice)

In verse I.13, Patañjali tells us that: "*tatra sthitau yatno' bhyāsaḥ*," "In this context, the effort to abide in (the cessation of identification with the fluctuations of consciousness) is a constant practice". This "effort to abide" in this higher state of consciousness manifests through the practice of various techniques, which include asanas, breathing, mudras, meditation and mantras.

But how should we practice? He further qualifies the types of practices required in verse I.14: "*sa tu dīrgha-kāla-nairantarya-satkāra-āsevito dṛḍha-bhūmiḥ.*" "However, this (practice only becomes) firmly established when properly and consistently attended to over a long (period of) time."

The natural tendency of the mind is to flow outwards towards sensory experiences. The purpose of this practice is to establish a counter habit of inward mindedness. In our modern, materialistic culture, we are constantly bombarded by the media with things to attract our attention, so we miss what is essential, the Self, our only lasting source of delight. This should serve as a warning to all who seek a quick, effortless route to enlightenment or a blissful hereafter. So often novices look for the "easy path" or the "quickest route." Our negative habits of mind are too firmly entrenched in most cases, to permit anything but a long, diligent process.

"Firmly established" means that one has established a habit of witnessing life's passing subjective and objective experiences. This can occur only when we practice for a long time, with devotion and faith in the results. It means integrating our spiritual life with our mundane life. If one doubts the efficacy of the practice or does it in a half hearted way, one cannot easily bring it into daily life.

These verses shed light on what qualifies as "tapas", "intense practice," and they indicate that it reflects no particular technique, but a way of practicing. "Tapas" means literally "straightening by fire", and the yogic literature is filled with stories of how intensive yogic practice has lead practitioners beyond their limitations.

"*Svadhyaya*" or "self-study" means the use of ones higher faculty, including the intellect, to know ones Self. It may include study of the sacred scriptures, mantra repetition, or observation of the psycho-dynamics of the mind. What was then a subjective experience can become objective, and one can distinguish more easily what is the personality and what is the Self. This leads to Self mastery.

"*Ishvara pranidhanani*" or surrender to the Supreme Being means cultivating unconditional love through bhakti or devotion, seeing the Lord everywhere. One forgets the ego's petty concerns and develops universal love. Surrender also implies letting go of what disturbs the mind, ("let go and let God"). The form of the Lord one chooses is a matter of personal choice. However, it is not an alternative to practice and detachment, but a component of them.

"*Vairagya*" (Detachment)

In verse I.2, right at the beginning of his text, Patañjali defines the initial phase of the Yoga process as "*yogaś-citta-vṛtti-nirodhaḥ,*" that is, "Yoga is the cessation of (identifying with) the fluctuations (arising within) consciousness". This provides us with the reason for the cultivation of detachment.

The word "*citta*" means consciousness and the term "*cittar*" (or Siddha) is the Tamil name for one who is a master of consciousness, or "one who is supremely conscious". It is the localized manifestation of "cit" or Absolute consciousness. While Patañjali does not define the term "*citta,*" its meaning can be determined from the contexts in which it appears in the *Yoga-Sūtras.* According to verse IV.23, consciousness is colored by the Self and the manifestations of Nature, the Seer and the Seen. This apparent and mistaken identification of the Self with the manifestations of nature (the Seen) is the cause of human suffering and the fundamental problem of human consciousness. As the *cittars* (tam.) have stated: "We are dreaming with our eyes open," because we identify not with who we are but with what we are not, ie. our dreams. It is a complete reversal of the true relationship between the Self and the fluctuations arising within consciousness. The Self is the pure, absolute subject, and is experienced as "I am." But in ordinary human consciousness, the Self has become an object: "myself," a personality, an ego ridden collection of thoughts, feelings and sensations which assumes the role of the subject. The habit of identifying with our thoughts, emotions, sensations, that is, egoism, is the nearly universal disease of ordinary human consciousness. The fluctuations (*vritti*) arising within consciousness, enumerated and explained in verse 1.5 to 1.11 such as "means of acquiring true knowledge," "misconception," "conceptualisation," "sleep" and "memory" must be cleansed of egoism, the strong habit of feeling "I am this emotion," "I am this memory," "I am this sensation," by the systematic cultivation of detachment, wherein one realizes "I am conscious of this emotion, memory, sensation and I am not this emotion, memory, sensation."

It is not the elimination of the fluctuations of consciousness themselves which will restore one's realization of the Self as one's identity. Were that the case, only the ultimate cessation of these movements, death, could bring about Self Realization. Self Realization would not be possible while living. As long as the world exists, there will always be fluctuations. What is problematic here is the habitual confusion "I am" (the Self) with "I am (the object of consciousness, emotion, memory, sensation)." What one must realize is that one may have thoughts, emotions, sensations, sleep, etc., but that one is not the thoughts, emotions, sensations, sleep, etc.

What is consciousness? While Patañjali does not define the term "*citta*," its meaning can be determined from the contexts in which it appears in Siddha literature. According to the Siddha Tirumūlar, a contemporary of Patañjali, who wrote "*Tirumandiram*"(4) verse 119:

> Our intelligence entangled in the senses
> Finds itself in very deep waters
> But inside our consciousness is a deeper
> Consciousness
> Which the Supreme Grace stimulates.

and Verse 122:

> Sivayoga is to know the Cit-Acit
> And for the Yoga-Penance qualify
> Self light becoming Self
> To enter undeviating, His lordly domain
> He granted me this - Nandi of the Nine Yoga.

Cit = The self-knowledge of Shiva consciousness
Acit = The ignorance of the Jiva, the soul or individualized spirit which upholds the living being.

(Patañjali is referred to twice in *Tirumandiram*, in verse 67 and 2790, see reference 4)

Contemporary Yoga has emphasized various techniques of Yoga, but too often ignored the need for "detachment." At its worst, Yoga today has become attached to the "performance" or "achievement" of various states, particularly in schools of hatha Yoga. This may be largely attributed to the values of our modern material culture, with emphasis on individualism, competition and attachment to material things or persons (as in "I love you," that is "I need you").

So why should contemporary practitioners of Yoga value Patañjali's teaching of detachment? In the first chapter of the *Yoga-Sūtras*,

Patañjali explains how an individual, in normal ordinary human consciousness, identifies with various mental movements or modifications, and states that they are "afflicted" or "non-afflicted." He identifies these in verse I.6 as means of acquiring true knowledge, misconception, conceptualization, sleep and memory. "Yoga is the cessation from (identifying with) the fluctuation (arising within) consciousness." (verse I.2) This process results ultimately in Self realization. "The Seer (Self) abides in his own true form." (verse I.3)

In verses I.15 and I.16 Patañjali distinguishes the preliminary and highest forms of detachment:

> I.15 "*dṛṣṭa-ānuśravika-viṣaya-vitṛṣṇasya vaśīkāra-saṁjñā vairāgyam,*" "Detachment is the emblem of the mastery of one who sees and hears an object without craving."

Detachment involves letting go, not of the objects which inhabit our world, but of the desire or craving to possess them, of the attachment, or need for them. We ignorantly confuse our source of happiness, our Self, with such objects, ignoring the true inner source of unconditional bliss. "Craving" is imagining how desirable something would be if one possessed it. Such illusions color our perceptions: one sees what one desires, not the reality, like someone looking into a mirror covered with dirt, fails to see the reality.

In the preliminary stage of detachment, one reminds oneself to release, to let go of this craving. Even the practice of the Yoga postures was originally intended for this purpose: to relax, let go of the tension, disease and discomfort of the physical body. There are many techniques to help remind oneself including various forms of meditation and mantras. Patañjali indicates two types of objects to detach from: objects of the external world, and "revealed" or "heard about" things which are described in sacred texts, such as heavenly states. "The emblem of the mastery" implies a detachment which is firmly established and integrated in all parts of ones life; one does not flee the world; one remains in it, but transcendental to it; one is continually conscious of a higher Reality.

In verse I.16: "*tat-paraṁ puruṣa-khyāter-guṇa-vaitṛṣṇyam,*" "That freedom from desire (activated by) the constituent forces (of Nature) (which arises) due to an individual's (Self) realization is supreme."

The ordinary person is involved in desires, activated by the forces of nature, with little or not control and only fleeting experiences of happiness. However, realizing the Self, the joy and peace is so fulfilling that automatically one gains discrimination between the Self and the non-Self. With this one loses desire for involvement even in subconscious motivated desires, memories and fantasies. It is detachment not based upon control, but on the spontaneous and constant awareness of one's greater Self, all pervasive and ever joyful.

The cultivation of detachment does not include pushing things away, nor encouraging them. During meditation it is characterized by a state of calmness, which allows one to be present with whatever comes up from the subconscious. Being present with something implies realizing "I am" rather than identifying with whatever emotion, memory or sense perception happens to be invading one's consciousness. It implies being a witness rather than allowing consciousness to be absorbed by objects of attention.

In verses I.30 Patañjali lists nine distractions of consciousness which are obstacles to cultivating the inner awareness of the Self:

> "*yādhi-styāna-saṁśaya-pramāda-ālasya-avirati-bhrānti-darśana-alabdha-bhūmikatva-anavasthitatvāni citta-vikṣepās-te' ntarāyāḥ,*" "Disease, dullness, doubt, carelessness, laziness, sense indulgence, false perception, failure to reach firm ground and instability - these distractions of consciousness are the obstacles."

The obstacles to inner awareness or witnessing are the distractions listed here. However they are not insurmountable. Through the repetition of mantras and other yogic sadhanas they may be overcome.

Too often, modern practitioners of Yoga find excuses for not continuing or intensifying their practice. Without recognizing the above distractions, how can one avoid being carried away by them.

Or, without recognizing what one is not, how can one recognize what one is? Our sadhana is to make this distinction, constantly, from moment to moment.

In verse I.31 he lists four emotional accompaniments to these obstacles:

> "*duḥkha-daurmanasya-aṅgam-ejayatva-śvāsa-praśvāsā vikṣepa-sahabhuvaḥ,*" "Accompaniments to the mental distractions include trembling in the body, unsteady inhalation (of the breath), depression and anxiety."

The mental distractions are those movements which cause us to forget or lose inner awareness. When we become very absorbed by our thoughts and lose our equilibrium, there may even be side effects in our emotions, like despair, anxiety, agitation in the physical body, or absence of calm, even breathing. Such accompaniments may serve to remind us just how far we have lost sight of our true Nature and thus help us to return to it. We can chant or do loving actions to change our emotions, or breathe deeply or do postures to quiet the mind, emotions and body. Psychological treatments are generally palliative and symptomatic, but such yogic activities go to the real causal part of our nature. The body-mind has a will and a memory of its own which was well-known in ancient times. A wholistic approach such as Yoga will prevent such accompaniments from creating major illnesses.

By regularly noting the presence of these nine distractions and their emotional accompaniments in our lives, we can gradually detach from and ultimately master them. In verses II.33 Patañjali recommends: "When disturbed by negative thoughts, opposite (positive) ones should be thought of." By cultivating through auto-suggestion and affirmations their opposites we enlist the subconscious in the process.

In verses I.32-39 he indicates various methods of concentration, meditation and breath control to develop undisturbed mental calmness and to prevent these obstacles and their accompaniments from arising.

Students of Babaji's Kriya Yoga can easily recognize its similarities with Patañjali's Kriya Yoga. Babaji and Patañjali were contemporaries, and had a common *paramguru*, "Nandi," so this is not surprising.

After delineating a great many "*siddhis*" or yogic miraculous powers which the *yogin* may develop as a result of intensive practice of Yoga, Patañjali advises us to detach even from them in verse III.50: "*tad-vairāgyād-api doṣa-bīja-kṣaye kaivalyam*," "Through detachment even towards [the *siddhis* of omniscience and omnipotence with] the destruction of the seed of this obstacle, there arises absolute freedom". So often we encounter what has been referred to as "spiritual materialism," that is, the power to do extraordinary or miraculous things, such as levitation, clairvoyance, astral travel, materialisation of objects. Patañjali wisely counsels us never to become attached to any of our attainments, even the greatest of yogic powers, for only the absolute, will satisfy us absolutely! Why settle for anything less?

In conclusion, while Patañjali cites various specific practices of Yoga, such as asanas, pranayam, and meditation, he does not emphasize any particular techniques. This is consistent with the culture of the Siddhas, wherein the highest teachings were shared only in person, and never written down. These supreme teachings were crystallized in the form of "kriyas," or "techniques to be practiced rigorously" and they were imparted only during initiation sessions. During such sessions the kriyas are both revealed and practiced under the supervision of the teacher. The kriyas were not written down so that only those who practiced them regularly could remember them. Thus the tradition of the Siddhas has been handed down orally to this day by an unbroken line of sincere practioners. All have their place in an integrated process. Patañjali tells us of the obstacles and how to overcome them: the mental distractions and emotional accompaniments, the attractions of powers, but lays emphasis above all on the means to overcome them: constancy of practice and detachment, "*abhyāsa*" and "*vairāgya*." This should remind us of two very important attitudes to maintain at all times, not simply on our meditation pillows or asana mats!

The writings the Siddhas are characteristically succinct and often difficult to understand for the non-initiate. This is particularly difficult for contemporary western students of Yoga who have had little or no contact with India, the homeland of Yoga, with its rich spiritual and philosophical traditions. So, the writings of the Yoga Siddhas may be understood on two different levels: that of the non-initiate and that of the initiate. In making this commentary, I have often referred to specific Kriyas, which initiates of Babaji's Kriya Yoga will recognize, in order to facilitate their understanding. Babaji derived his Kriya Yoga from the teachings of the 18 Siddha tradition, which includes Siddha Patañjali. His Kriya Yoga is an elaborate system, which synthesizes and crystallizes their teachings. By understanding the philosophical sources of Babaji's Kriya Yoga, I believe that contemporary students will be able to appreciate the purpose of the techniques to a much greater degree. May this commentary inspire everyone to apply themselves intensely and continuously to the practice of Yoga.

Chapter 1: SAMĀDHI-PĀDA

This first chapter (*pāda),* provides some of the most important concepts about the process of *Yoga* and its results. Cognitive absorption (s*amādhi)* is such a result, and Patañjali brings us to a clear understanding of just what it is towards the end of this first chapter. As *Yoga* is a scientific art, a progressive system, Patañjali leads us through it much the same way an engineer might point out the features of a blue print. While he does not teach us how to perform specific practices, his blueprint will indicate in fair detail how they all fit together and what the results will resemble. The succinct form of the *sūtras,* like the engineers blueprints, are not to be confused with the reality, which they symbolize. Indian writers in general, and fully accomplished *yogins* (*siddhas)* like Patañjali and Tirumūlar specifically, realized the limitations of language, and used words in a suggestive manner. They wished to point to a deeper reality, which could not be grasped with mere words. Their works were often written in such a way so as to deliberately obscure the meaning from the non-initiate. A good grasp of the concepts revealed in this introductory chapter will enable the reader to understand what follows in the subsequent chapters, in which the processes and results of *Yoga* are described in much greater detail.

1. *atha-yoga-anuśāsanam*

atha = now

yoga = union

anuśāsanam = exposition

Now [begins] the exposition on y*oga.*

The term *atha* or now is a word used to call the readers attention to the beginning of an important treatise.

2. *yogaś-citta-vṛtti-nirodhaḥ*

yoga = Yoga

citta-vṛttiḥ = fluctuations of consciousness

nirodhaḥ = cessation

Yoga is the cessation [of identifying with] the fluctuations [arising within] consciousness.

Here it is appropriate to first explain some of the oldest concepts in Indian metaphysical thought: the term nature (*prakṛti*) and Self (*puruṣa*) in verses I.16, 24. *Prakṛti* is everything besides the Self and includes the entire cosmos from the material to the psychic levels. Unlike the Self (I am....), which is purely subjective, *prakṛti* is objective reality, that which is observed by the Self. It is real, however transitory it may be. *Puruṣa,* the Self, is pure subject, at the core of consciousness. It illuminates the consciousness. Without it, the mind and psyche would have no conscious activity, just as a light bulb without invisible electricity would radiate no light. *Prakṛti* exists as nature in its transcendental, undefined state as well as its multiform, differentiated manifestations. This Self is to be distinguished from the self of the limited personality and body. Sometimes, one refers to the true Self, as that eternal being at the core of everyone, the *atman,* or *jiva,* as opposed to the little self, the person or personality, the sum of our memories and limited identifications held together by egoism.

The word *citta,* consciousness and the term *cittar* (pronounced *siddhar*) is the Tamil word for one who is a master of consciousness. It is the localized manifestation of Absolute Consciousness *(cit).* While Patañjali does not define the term consciousness (*citta*) its meaning can be determined from the contexts in which it appears in the Sūtras. According to verse IV.23, consciousness is colored by the Self and the manifestations of nature, the Seer and the Seen. This apparent and mistaken identification of the Self, or Seer, with the manifestations of Nature (the Seen) is the cause of human suffering and the fundamental problem of human consciousness. As the *cittars (tam.)* have stated: "We are dreaming with our eyes open because we identify not with who we are, but with what we are not, our dreams." It is a complete reversal of the true relationship between the Self and objects of consciousness. The Self has become an object and myself, the personality, an ego-ridden collection of thoughts, feelings and sensations has taken on the role of the subject. The habit of identifying with our thoughts, emotions, sensations, that is, egoism, is the disease of human consciousness. The fluctuations (*vṛttiḥ*) arising within consciousness, enumerated and explained in verse I.5 to I.11, such as the means of acquiring true knowledge, misconceptions, conceptualization, sleep and memory must be cleansed of egoism, the strong habit of feeling, "I am this emotion," "I am this memory," "I am this sensation," by the systematic cultivation of detachment, wherein one realizes "I am conscious of this emotion, memory, sensation and I am not this emotion, memory, sensation."

In *Babaji's Kriya Yoga*, the first meditation technique, *śuddhi dhyāna kriyā*, has this change in perspective (or - change in consciousness) as its purpose. Like all habits, egoism lives in the subconscious level of the mind, that is, the part that is below our normal everyday realm of awareness. This level is, however, accessible through the various methods of *Yoga*.

It is not the elimination of the modifications of consciousness that will restore one's realization of the Self as one's identity. As long as the world exists, there will always be modifications. What is problematic here is the habitual confusion of "I am" (the Self) with "I am" (the object of consciousness, emotion, memory, sensation).

What is consciousness? The meaning of consciousness (*citta*) can be determined from the context in which it appears in Siddha literature. According to Tirumūlar:

> Our intelligence entangled in the senses,
> Finds itself in very deep waters,
> But inside our consciousness is a deeper
> Consciousness.
> Which the Supreme Grace stimulates. (TM 119)

and Verse 122:

> *Śivayoga* is to know the *cit-acit*
> And for the *yoga-penance* qualify;
> Self-light becoming Self,
> To enter undeviating, His lordly domain;
> He granted me this - *Nandi* of the Nine *Yogas*.

cit = The Self-knowledge of *Śiva*-consciousness.
acit = The ignorance of the, the soul or individualized spirit which upholds the living being.

Practice: As various disturbing thoughts, emotions, or sensations arise, ask the question: "Could I let it go?" Cultivate detachment towards them.

3. *tadā draṣṭuḥ sva-rūpe' vasthānam*

tadā = then

draṣṭuḥ = the Seer

svarūpe = in one's own form

a*vasthānam* = abides

Then the Seer abides in his own true form.

"Then" implies that what follows is a consequence of the process of purifying the habit of identifying with the fluctuations arising within consciousness, described in the preceding verse. What follows is a permanent state of Self-realization, not a temporary experience, which can be dispersed by the waves of mental distractions. In ordinary physical consciousness, one habitually identifies with mental forms and emotions. By the practice of such meditation techniques as ś*uddhi dhyāna kriyā* or *mantras,* one may develop a profound sense of detachment. The "Seer" is the Self. At the end of the process of *Yoga,* the individual soul (*jīva*), realizes that it is "*Śiva*", the Supreme Lord. The individual soul (*jīva*) assumes, by expansion, its true nature or form (*Śiva*) and no longer identifies with the lower physical or mental vehicles.

According to Tirumūlar:

In this *turiyatita jagrat* state,
The Lord Of Dance with *jīva* in union stands
When that union takes place *māyā* vanishes away
That very day *jīva* attains *Śiva* form. (TM 2277)

"*Jagrat*" refers to the waking state; "*turiya*" *is* the fourth state of consciousness, beyond waking, dreaming and deep sleep; super consciousness *(turiyatita)* means beyond *turiya).*

Practice: Repeat: "Now nothing can disturb me anymore" often, as an autosuggestion, particularly before going to sleep or when coming out of meditation.

4. *vṛtti-sārūpyam-itaratra*

vṛtti(ḥ) = fluctuations of consciousness

sārūpyam = assimilation; conformity; identification

itaratra = otherwise

Otherwise, there is an identification [by the individuated self] with the fluctuations [of consciousness].

In the state of ordinary human consciousness, the individual identifies with all of his or her mental and emotional movements, which arise for the most part, from the subconscious mind. If you ask another person: "Who are you?" typically he or she will reply that he is Mr. X or that she is Miss Y, their profession, sex, religion, family or even who their employer is, or what they love most in the world. But all of these identifications are only thoughts, based upon memory. It is indeed rare to find someone who identifies with his or her true Self, the *ātman* as the *yogins* say. In this essential Self, there is no difference between you and I. By the practice of *śuddhi dhyāna kriyā,* one gradually detaches from these fictional identifications.

"Otherwise" implies that Self-remembrance is not constant. In ceasing to identify with what one is not, there are times when one forgets. In confusion we identify with a current dominant emotion, like anger - a sensation, like fatigue - or thoughts, like judgments or memories. We should develop detachment and remain vigilant so as to prevent the mind from obscuring the underlying Pure Self-Consciousness. The practice of all forms of *Yoga* can aid Self-remembrance of realization.

Practice: Remember the inner Self, which always remains in a state of equanimity, which lies behind all experiences, like string, holding the necklace of beads together.

5. *vṛttayaḥ pañcatayaḥ kliṣṭa-akliṣṭāḥ*

vṛttayaḥ = fluctuations arising within consciousness

pañca-taya = five-fold

kliṣṭāḥ = afflicted

akliṣāḥ = non-afflicted

The fluctuations [of consciousness] are five-fold, being afflicted and non-afflicted.

In the beginning it is not always possible to abide in the consciousness of the Self because we are in the habit of allowing our consciousness to become completely involved in the objects of attention.

Discrimination (*viveka),* is an important practice to be done at all times. It will set the stage for meditation (*dhyāna),* which is continuous reflection on a particular object and cognitive absorption (*samādhi*).

Patañjali classifies fluctuations of consciousness (*citta-vṛttiḥ)* as afflicted versus unafflicted, not painful versus pleasurable. Afflicted modifications involve ego, false identification, contraction of awareness and selfishness; non-afflicted thoughts involve selflessness, pure love and expansion of awareness, interiorization and Self-realization.

Each of the five types of fluctuations (*vṛttiḥ*) can be afflicted or non-afflicted. For example, sleep can be afflicted when one is identified with the dreams or the body. Sleep can be non-afflicted as in the practice of *yoga nidrā,* when one remains aware, even while the body takes rest. (This *Yoga* is taught in *Babaji's Kriya Yoga* level II initiation).

We become troubled by thoughts and feelings when we do not practice discrimination towards fluctuations of consciousness (*citta-vṛttiḥ)* which are selfish and which lead to suffering. This is also why activities of selfless service (*karma yoga),* help us overcome selfishness and consequently, our own suffering.

Afflicted thoughts involve desires, which if not satisfied lead to frustration, and if satisfied, bring fear of loss and further desire. When we are not satisfied by what we get, (whatever it may be), a vicious circle can arise of chasing chimerical desire-filled objects or situations. Our sense of well-being, which is an inner state, is falsely associated with outer things or circumstances. We fear losing something or suffering from what may or may not happen. We often imagine that the fulfillment of some desire will give us lasting happiness. Unafflicted thoughts, for example, contemplating a sunset, leave us with a feeling of peace.

Practice: As you go through your days watch your thoughts carefully. Notice how thoughts perpetuate attachments and aversions. Write down all the thoughts you have which are afflicted. At the same time sit back and say to yourself: "Mind, I want you to be peaceful and happy; consciously release those thoughts which disturb your peace."

Remember, you are not what you think (the process is not so much about realizing, as it is about staying realized).

6. *pramāṇa-viparyaya-vikalpa-nidrā-smṛtayaḥ*

pramāṇam = means of acquiring knowledge

viparyaya = misconception

vikalpa = conceptualisation, imagination

nidrā = sleep, slumber

smṛti = memory; recollection

These five are: the means of acquiring true knowledge, misconception, conceptualization, sleep and memory.

Here Patañjali names the five types of *vṛttis* (fluctuations of consciousness) and in the following verses explains them one after another. Patañjali has distinguished the different types in order to help us cease to identify with them.

7. *pratyakṣa-anumāna-āgamāḥ pramāṇāni*

pratyakṣa = perception via the five senses

anumāna = inference; reflection

āgamāḥ = sacred works

pramāṇāni = means of obtaining true knowledge

The means of obtaining true knowledge are: perception via the five senses, inference and the study of sacred works.

As we will find it more difficult to remove false identification with all the types of fluctuations of consciousness simultaneously, it is better to distinguish them and to use the means of obtaining right knowledge (*pramāṇāni*) to help us become aware of the other types of fluctuations of consciousness (*cittavṛttiḥ*) such as conceptualization (*vikalpa*), misconception (*viparyaya*), sleep (*nidrā*) and memory (*smṛti*).

True knowledge should help us in our mental "house cleaning." To let go of false identification with the feeling "I am" what I see, hear, taste, touch, smell, infer, or have received testimony about, we must remove egoism. So we should know the means of obtaining true knowledge (*pramāṇāni*), and be aware when we have found it.

Direct perception or perception via the five senses (*pratyakṣa*) is what we validate by personal experience. This is why the scientific approach is emphasized with respect to the techniques, which are viewed as hypotheses to be tested in the laboratory of one's own consciousness.

Inference (*anumāna*) is another source. An example of inference is: "Where there is smoke, there must be fire." It infers the cause from the effect. Another example is: Relief of constipation after doing postures, which massage the intestines, can enable one to infer that the postures contributed to the relief! From a feeling of peace after meditation we can infer that the meditation was authentic and done well.

Scriptural testimony from sacred works (*āgamāḥ*) is the recording of sages and prophets who have perceived the Truth, and which has been handed down since ancient times by others who have found it to be effective. While it may appear in different forms of presentation, its essence is the same. It is important to validate what you believe, perceive or infer against the teachings of the scriptures, because there may be surprising long-term effects which you may not perceive in the short run. You should not believe something or someone blindly. Refer to scriptural authorities. If you find the teaching there also, you may follow it as a tried and true method. This is important in a time when many are teaching things which they have created, based upon limited experience, or which are adaptations or even radical modifications of tried and true methods.

Practice: Practice direct perception via the five sense faculties (*pratyakṣa)*: Let go of judgments, notions, and beliefs about anything. Allow yourself to have no opinion, no knowledge about anything for a day. Eat, drink, see, and read as if you are tasting life for the first time. Allow direct perception (*pratyakṣa)* to suggest the description and quality of what you experience. Let everything be as it is without reacting to anything.

Practice of inference (*anumāna)*: Allow the intellect to consider the chain of cause and effect between events.

Relying on the sacred works (*āgamāḥ)* of the sages: Read daily from the scriptures of your choice on topics related to the path out of suffering (*dharma)* and of the nature of reality (*satya)* and metaphysics.

8. *viparyayo mithyā-jñānam-atad-rūpa-pratiṣṭham*

viparyaya = misconception

mithyā = false

jñāna = knowledge

a-tadrūpa = not on that form

pratiṣṭham = based on

Misconception is false knowledge not based upon it's true form.

Misconception begins with an external objective stimulus. Most of our experience is colored by our desires or fears - we see someone or experience some event and because of our prejudices or desires or attitudes we form conclusions, which are illusory. If we want to see things as they are, we need to let go of our attachment to such misconceptions as racism, envy, jealousy, lust, and all fears and desires both great and small.

Examples of misconception (*viparyaya*) or illusions, are judgments made about someone based upon their skin color, becoming infatuated with a beautiful woman or a handsome man, a mirage in the distance, a rope on the floor mistakenly perceived as a snake, or mistaking someone in a crowd for an acquaintance.

A-tadrūpa refers back to verse I.3, the realization of one's true form (*svarūpa)* that which is really there, in essence. When we base our judgments upon what is imagined, feared or desired, we suffer from misconceptions.

Practice: Make a list of your prejudices and desires. Be aware of them, so that the moment they pop up in your life, you can change the way you see them. Notice how often they continue to appear, and how you finally change the way you see them.

9. *śabda-jñāna-anupātī vastu-śūnyo vikalpaḥ*

śabda = verbal communication; sound ;language

jñāna = knowledge

anupātī = following; consequence

vastu = object; real abiding substance

śūnya = void; without, having none

vikalpa = imagination, conceptualization

Conceptualization is the result of knowledge [acquired from] verbal communication having no real abiding substance.

Conceptualization (*vikalpa*) includes the thoughts, and ideas, which flow through the mind as in daydreaming or abstract thinking. It does not need any objective external object to stimulate it. It is the incessant commentary of the mind talking to itself, and so, is said to flow from what can be put into words. Mentally thinking about our experience, because it never stops, prevents us from experiencing reality as it is. However, it is not entirely useless, as it may lead us to a means of silencing itself wherein we can experience the transcendental Self.

Our mind tells us something and we believe it. It has nothing to do with the truth. We get caught up in a thought and it becomes like a monster in our mind. It disturbs our peace. We are unable to experience what is actually happening due to this creation in our mind. One must learn to quiet the mind.

Practice: Practice *śuddhi dhyāna kriyā.* Abide in the peace of the Self. Rest, and watch any thoughts which arise, coming from outside, passing through the space of the mind, and leaving without a trace. Feel the Divine Presence within yourself. Let the Divine swallow the thought monster in rapturous silence.

10. *abhāva-pratyaya-ālambanā vṛttir-nidrā*

abhāva = nothingness, non-existence

pratyaya = thought, notion, belief

ālambana = support

vṛttiḥ = fluctuation [of consciousness]

nidrā = sleep

The fluctuation of sleep is based on a belief in non-existence.

During deep sleep there is only the thought of nothingness. If one has other thoughts it is in the dream state. There are four states: physical consciousness, dream state (in daydreaming or in sleep), deep dreamless sleep and the fourth state (*turya),* which is pure consciousness - unclouded by any thoughts, even by the belief that there is "nothing" in deep sleep. In *turya* the consciousness does not withdraw, but transcends the subject-object duality, in the other three states. In sleep (*nidrā),* the consciousness first turns inwards, away from outward sounds and sensations, then gradually it turns away from even thoughts and dreams. At its climax it turns away from everything except the one experience of "nothingness". After a deep sleep, upon awaking, one remembers that one was conscious only of the "nothingness".

Practice: Before you go to sleep, when you get into bed, simply think of the Divine. Think of sleep as a time for you to reach into Consciousness. Wake up without use of an alarm clock as often as possible. When you awaken in the morning, keep still. Do not even move your head. Teach your body to remain still, suspended between sleep and waking, with a very tranquil will to remember. If you sometimes remember a word or a gesture, a color or an image, hang onto it and don't move. You will build a bridge between these two mental modifications. Do not be in a hurry to get up. Think of the Divine.

Practice: The practice of *yoga nidrā* taught during the *Anthar Kriya Yoga* spiritual retreat brings about the experience of *turya.* The first meditation technique *śuddhi dhyāna kriyā* helps one to remove the feeling of "I am the one sleeping" within the subconscious mind, preparing one for the experience of *turya.*

11. *anubhūta-viṣaya-asaṁpramoṣaḥ smṛtiḥ*

anubhūta = experienced

viṣaya(ḥ) = object

asaṁpramoṣaḥ = not forgotten

smṛtiḥ = memory

Memory is not letting an object experienced be carried away [from one's consciousness].

Memory *(smṛtiḥ)* includes the recall of experiences through the five senses, as well as through concepts or ideas. Memory is a function of desire. We tend to remember our likes and dislikes. Our manner of filtering our present experience and of creating associations between our experience and our memories reflects this.

Memories are generally in two categories: Those remembered voluntarily, and those remembered involuntarily. The latter are usually stimulated by associations with present experiences and fueled by desire-laden emotions, which are stored in the subconscious. Memories and desire-emotions constitute the samskaras or subconscious tendencies, which drive us. *Yoga* involves cleansing one's consciousness of subconscious impressions (*saṁskāras)* through detachment (*vairāgya)* and living more and more consciously in the present. Through detachment these desires and subsconsious impressions (*saṁskāras)* lose their force. Memory becomes more and more of the voluntary type. All phases and techniques in *Kriya Yoga* contribute to this purification and increasing awareness.

Practice: Be childlike. See everything as if you are seeing it for the first time. Practice being aware as you do each thing. Learn and practice the *jnanbaha kriya shangali korvai (tam.)* Memory Chain *kriyā* from the *Babaji's Kriya Yoga* Level III initiation, and explore memories from throughout your life and previous lives.

12. *abhyāsa-vairāgyābhyāṁ tan-nirodhaḥ*

abhyāsa = by constant, repeated practice

vairāgya = by detachment

tan = these

nirodhaḥ = cease; here: cease to identify with (see verse I.2)

By constant practice and with detachment [arises] the cessation [of identifying with the fluctuations of consciousness].

Here Patañjali prescribes the most important method in Kriya Yoga (see verses I.2 and II.1) for the cleansing of egoism which comes from identifying with the fluctuations arising within consciousness.

By constant practice (*abhyāsa)* refers to concentrating on what one is, the Self, or in preparatory exercises, on objects of concentration (as it is easier to concentrate on an object than on the formless Absolute). Detachment (*vairāgya)* refers to ceasing to identify with that which we are not - the passing thoughts, emotions that are sense or memory based. As the practitioner lets go of those movements, which have been suppressed in the subconscious mind, through such techniques as *śuddhi dhyāna kriyā* or through the repetition of sacred seed syllables (*bīja mantras*), what is left is pure consciousness, i.e. the Self, becomes manifest. Constant practice is like a person bailing out a small sinking boat. If we stop focusing on that pure conscious Self, we are overwhelmed by the strong habitual pull of egoism, just as if one stops bailing the boat they become overwhelmed by the in-rushing water. Constant practice means remembering the Supreme absolute in the midst of all changes and passing show.

<u>Practice</u>: (1) Maintain the perspective of the Self within, witnessing everything. Cultivate the Self, the awareness and feeling of the inner Divinity. Become established in It. Feel its beauty permeating every experience. (2) Allow thoughts and emotions to come, and go, without disturbing this perspective. Let go when there is attachment to them. (3) Learn and practice *śuddhi dhyāna kriyā* and the other *dhyāna kriyas* to close or open the Nine Openings of the human body, as taught in *Babaji's Kriya Yoga* Level III teachings.

13. *tatra sthitau yatno' bhyāsaḥ*

tatra = under these circumstances

sthitau = remaining or abiding in

yatna = effort

a*bhyāsa* = constant, repeated practice

In this context, the effort to abide in [the cessation of identification with the fluctuations of consciousness] is a constant practice.

Steadiness of mind is acquired by the practice of the various *kriyās* including yogic postures (*āsanas*), breath control (*prāṇāyāma*), hand positions (*mudrās*), meditation (*dhyāna*) and *mantras*. The first techniques of meditation in *Babaji's Kriya Yoga* are particularly important so that the mind does not get carried away with thoughts and lost in identification with sensory things. By maintaining a witness consciousness in the midst of all changes, one can develop a constant sense of one's true Self.

Typically, the mind is not steady, but constantly flitting about from one thing to another, often chaotically. It is like a homeless dog, wandering everywhere. In the beginning, it resists the direction of "the master," just as such a untrained dog would resist or ignore instructions during its first day of dog training school. Training the mind to be steady is not unlike training a dog to obey in dog training school. It will not be effective to beat the dog, or to get discouraged if it does not obey initially. What is needed are clear, steady, persistent commands to the mind, and much patience. Gradually the "dog-mind" will begin to realize that now it has a "master," and will obey. Too often, the beginning student does not realize how much patience is required, and easily becomes discouraged. Be gentle with the "dog-mind," but firm and persistent.

Patañjali says that the practice should be constant and not just for a few minutes a day. During the retreats, one learns techniques and a lifestyle, which assists us in maintaining this awareness 24 hours a day, even during sleep and daily activities. Practice is *sādhana* (literally, "the means for attainment") or remembrance of the Self. One's joy in life is directly proportional to the amount of *sādhana* that one performs.

Practice: Practice all of the *kriyās* skillfully, with full attention. Perform all actions with full awareness.

14. *sa tu dīrgha-kāla-nairantarya-satkāra-āsevito dṛḍha-bhūmiḥ*

sa = this

tu = but

dīrgha = long

kāla = time

nairantarya = without break, uninterruptedly

satkāra = kind treatment, honour, reverence

āsevita = well attended to

dṛḍha = firmly

bhūmiḥ = established; grounded; earth

However, this [practice only becomes] firmly established when properly and consistently attended to over a long [period of] time.

The natural tendency of the mind is to flow outwards towards sensory experience. Here, Patañjali tells us how to establish a counter habit of inward attentiveness. (see verse I.29)

Firmly established (*dṛḍha-bhūmiḥ)* means that the yogic consciousness becomes integrated into all the parts of our being, including its foundation, the subconscious, when it has been practiced for a long time, continually, with devotion and faith in its results. If one doubts its efficacy or does it in a half-hearted way, one cannot easily derive the results towards one's self.

How many people take to spirituality as an escape from the reality of daily life? When the yogic attention permeates our subconscious habits, it supports us in all activities, even during periods of stress and challenge. Techniques taught in the *Babaji*'s *Kriya Yoga* Level II initiation assist us to develop this constant awareness during daily activities and even during rest.

"Practice [becomes firmly established]" (*sa [abhyāsaḥ]...dṛḍha bhūmiḥ),* means that in all activities we maintain the perspective of the witness, the pure subject, as distinct from the objects of awareness.

As few persons initially have the motivation or the capacity to practice continuously and with intensity, it is preferable to begin by practicing at regular times each day, gradually increasing the length of time for each session. Soon, one may be able to find time for more sessions. At some point one begins to integrate the practice during activities of daily life. One should maintain an attitude of reverence (*satkāra)* towards one's practice. This may include making a lifetime commitment to the practice.

Practice: Do your *sādhana* with a sense of gratitude, reverence, joy and enthusiasm. These qualities will support a consistency of effort. Cultivate the inner Self- awareness constantly, and remain grounded in That throughout all of life's experiences. Learn and practice *nityānanda kriyā,* from the Babaji's Kriya Yoga Level II initiation

15. *dṛṣṭa-ānuśravika-viṣaya-vitṛṣṇasya vaśīkāra-saṁjñā vairāgyam*

dṛṣṭa = seen

ānuśravika = heard

viṣaya = object

vitṛṣṇasya = of the one without craving

vaśīkāra = mastery; accomplishment

saṁjñā = knowledge; sign, emblem

vairāgyam = detachment

Detachment is the emblem of the mastery of one who sees and hears an object without craving.

Here Patañjali defines detachment (*vairāgya).* Craving for objects seen or heard (*dṛṣṭa-ānuśravika-viṣaya*) arises from the subconscious and colors our perceptions - we see our desires rather than the Reality. Disassociation, or detachment from them, through the practice of *śuddhi dhyāna kriyā* and other techniques of *Yoga,* leads one to a state of non-attachment wherein one experiences the Self, and then lives selflessly, for others. In this state of deep peace, objects seen and heard pass like clouds, without disturbance. We remain attached only to the Self.

Detachment (*vairāgya)* means that there is no desire for the objects Seen or heard about - the latter refers to memories, or associations, which may arise when new stimuli occurs. It may also include things revealed in sacred texts, or in heavenly realms. Renunciation, or detachment, does not mean giving up objects but rather the craving (*tṛṣṇa*) or desire for them. Craving is imagining how desirable something would be if one possessed it. It is an illusion. Happiness exists inside our self, not in objects outside of our self. Detachment allows one to remain in the presence of our true Self. It is characterized by the feeling of calmness, despite the presence of many objects of attention or potential distractions. This calmness is the emblem of detachment and includes not only an outward passivity, but an inner equilibrium.

Mastery of detachment (*vairāgya)* begins with detachment towards objects experienced through the five senses. In their presence there is first an effort not to indulge in craving or desire for them. At a later stage, mastery (*vaśīkāra*) extends towards thoughts about sensuous enjoyment. One makes an effort to detach mental fantasies. Still later as the attachment becomes weaker, the detachment is nearly effortless in the waking state, but must still be applied towards subconscious tendencies, for example, through the practice of autosuggestion or affirmation.

Practice: Cultivate detachment and equanimity whether you receive praise or blame, experience success or failure, loss or gain, pleasure or pain, whether you are in the midst of many others or alone. Learn and practice *śuddhi dhyāna kriyā* and related techniques, integrating it into daily life occurrences or circumstances.

16. *tat-paraṁ puruṣa-khyāter-guṇa-vaitṛṣṇyam*

tad = that

paraṁ = supreme

puruṣa = Self; the individual

khyāteḥ = due to the realization

guṇa = constituent forces, attributes; quality

vaitṛṣṇyam = freedom

That freedom from the constituent forces [of nature] [which arises] due to an individual's [Self]-realization is supreme.

The ordinary person, who has not yet begun to practice *Yoga*, is involved in desires, which are activated by the three constituent forces of nature (*guṇas*) with little or no control and only fleeting glimpses of happiness. These are: the natural tendency towards activity (*rajas*); the tendency towards inertia (*tamas*), and the tendency towards balance (*sattva*). We are subject to much illusion, like someone looking at a distorted mirror. By the practice of yogic *sādhana*, peace of mind grows. We begin to gain some control over the desires and to cleanse the subconscious tendencies. There is some detachment from objects of desire, which were former sources of pain and pleasure. But we are still subject to their memory and consequently we frequently fantasize. At first, detachment requires effort.

However, when we permanently realize the Self, the joy and peace is so fulfilling that automatically we gain discrimination between the Self and the non-Self, and with this we lose desire for involvement even in subconscious motivated desires, memories and fantasies. They lose their force and wither away. It is desirelessness not based upon control but on the spontaneous and constant awareness of our greater Self, all pervasive and ever joyful, in all circumstances. Supreme detachment is effortless. The discriminative knowledge, which this latter stage of detachment brings, allows the *yogin* to see the limitations of all objects of desire. The resulting clarity of vision provides a steadiness in detachment, and enables lasting Self-realization.

Svāmi Hariharananda Aranya has made a very important point about this: "Man's knowledge is directly or indirectly conducive to the elimination of misery. That knowledge which brings about final and entire cessation of all sorrows is the highest form of knowledge. Then there cannot be anything higher to know." Regarding *para-vairāgya*, the *Kaṭha Upaniṣad* says: "The wise, knowing of the eternal bliss, do not look for the immutable in ephemeral things."(1)

Practice: Aspire to live in a state of equanimity, where you no longer identify with various desires, by cultivating detachment, contentment, endurance, fearlessness, cheerfulness and adaptability in all situations. If you just cannot feel this in any particular situation ask yourself "Why?" Only by truthfully answering this question will you gain permanent and effortless release from what keeps you from Self-realization.

17. *vitarka-vicāra-ānanda-asmitā-(rūpa-) anugamāt-saṁprajñātaḥ*

vitarka = observation; discursive thought

vicāra = reflection, discernment, exercise of reason

ānanda = rejoicing
asmitā = I-am-ness; awareness of the Self

rūpa = form

anugamāt = accompanied by; following

saṁprajñāta = distinguished, object-oriented, cognitive absorption

Distinguished [*saṁprajñāta*] cognitive absorption is accompanied by observation, reflecting, rejoicing and awareness of the Self.

In this verse, Patañjali begins a section, which discusses the various types of cognitive absorption (*samādhi).* This arises after we cease to identify with the five fluctuations arising within consciousness. In cognitive absorption (*samādhi),* one realizes pure subject awareness. Cognition is knowing (gnosis) particularity from within. In absorption, the object and the subject become identified. It is not a mere void. So the four accompaniments of this first type of *samādhi,* namely, of observation, reflection, rejoicing and the experience of "I-am," are not mere fluctuations of consciousness (*citta-vṛttiḥ*) as in verse I.6, but inspired products of this fusion between subject and object. Unlike non-distinguished cognitive absorption (*asaṁprajñāta samādhi)* (verse I.18), here there are material or subtle objects as supports or points of departure, which may be any of the forms of Nature, including the most sublime levels of transcendental existence. Some refer to this as "distinguished" *samādhi,* because the accompaniments involve distinctions.

With reference to the beginning of the commentary on verse I.2, to know *puruṣa* one must first understand *prakṛti.* The first step comes by contemplating nature in its various manifestations:

1. *Vitarka* = Observation and analysis of material nature, down to its elemental characteristics.

   Savitarka samādhi occurs when the mind is focused on an object in nature.

   Practice: Perform, concentration on and absorption in material objects (*trāṭaka kriyā),* or the meditation *kriyās* (*dhyāna kriyās)* involving the five sense faculties (*jñāna indriyas*).
2. *Vicāra* = Reflection on subtle nature experiencing the truth of abstractions, without reference to material observation.

Savicāra samādhi occurs when the mind is focused on an abstraction.

Practice: Practice the *dhyāna kriyās* involving abstract concepts such as truth, love, wisdom and mathematics.

3. *Ānanda* = Pure joy or bliss. Rejoicing, which is independent of outer circumstances, an accompaniment of cognitive absorption.

   Ānanda samādhi occurs when the mind is focused upon the experience of joy itself , beyond all abstractions.

   Practice: The technique of continual bliss (*nityānanda kriyā)* taught in *Babaji's Kriya Yoga* level III initiation.

4. *Asmitā* = I-am-ness. Pure subjectivity.

   Sâsmita samādhi occurs when you are only aware of "I am;" however the *saṁskāras,* or subconscious impressions are still buried in a seed form in the mind, and may manifest.

   Practice: *Sarvikalpa (*the Tamil equivalent of *saṁprajñātaḥ) samādhi kriyā* taught in *Babaji's Kriya Yoga* level III initiation. By practicing the *samādhi kriyās* in order, going inward from the gross to the most subtle, one can separate Self (*purusa*) from nature *prakriti.*

18. *virāma-pratyaya-abhyāsa-pūrvaḥ saṁskāra-śeṣo' nyaḥ*

virāma = cessation, detachment

pratyaya = thought, notion, experience, belief

abhyāsa = constant, repeated practice

pūrva = previous, formerly, aforementioned, preceded by
saṁskāra = subconscious impressions, habits, tendencies

śeṣo = residual, that which is spared, the rest

anya = other

Preceded by constant practice with the contemplation of detachment, [there is the] other [non-distinguished state of cognitive absorption, "*asaṁprajñāta samādhi*" which possesses] residual subconscious impressions.

Here there are no longer objective supports. After understanding *prakṛti,* nature in its four manifestations (material, subtle, pure joy, and I-am-ness) as described in the commentary of the previous verse, we may detach, or let go of it, and abide as the pure Self. It is a state wherein one transcends all accompanying manifestations of distinguished cognitive absorption *(prajñātaḥ).* Their cessation occurs only after constant and prolonged practice of detachment (as described in verse 12) through various methods. Non-distinguished cognitive absorption (*asaṁprajñāta samādhi)* follows distinguished cognitive absorption (*saṁprajñātaḥ samādhi)* and becomes possible only with a moment-to-moment practice of detachment and Self-awareness over many years. Supreme detachment (*paravairāgya)* is therefore the means to attain it, because it cannot be attained when an object is the basis of concentration. Only a latent impression of detachment itself remains.

In verses 2269 to 2295, *Tirumantiram* describes the ascent of *consciousness* through the realm of the five physical and subtle senses involved in nature, and beyond, through the higher states of experience (*parāvasthā*). This culminates in pure experience (*śudhhāvasthā)* which like the non-distinguished cognitive absorption (*asaṁprajñāta samādhi)* transcends all distinctions of object-subject duality.

The limited sphere of *tattvas*
Five times five
And *māyā* impure
Unreal are they
Leaving them,
Let *jīva* ascend,
Into the sphere of *mamaya* (Pure-Impure)
Penetrating it, further beyond,
In the state of *parāvasthā*
That is pure *(śuddha)*

There the Soul is All-Existence,
And Non-Existence at once. (TM 2294)

Practice: Continuously practice letting go of involvement and identification with all mental movements, using the various *kriyās* of *Babaji's Kriya Yoga,* particularly those taught during the level II initiation, until equanimity is established. Practice *nirvikalpa* (the Tamil equivalent of *asaṁprajñātaḥ) samādhi kriyā* as *Babaji's Kriya Yoga* level III initiation.

19. *bhava-pratyayo videha-prakṛti-layānām*

bhava = arisen or produced from, source, origin, existence,

pratyayaḥ = co-operating cause; notion, ground

videha = bodiless, incorporeal, disincarnate, formless

prakṛti-layānām = absorption in, clinging to, merged in na ture

Of those [*yogin's*] who [being] disincarnate are absorbed into nature [there is] the intention of becoming.

In the distinguished cognitive absorption *(saṁprajñātaḥ samādhi,* discussed in verse 17) the buried seeds (*bīja)* of desire can still come into the conscious mind given the proper opportunity, because of the presence of habitually patterned subconscious impressions *(saṁskāras)* in one's consciousness. If we die before attaining the highest state of *asaṁprajñātaḥ samādhi* (described in verse 18), a state of cognitive absorption undistinguished by any support, we go onto become formless *(videha) beings,* one of the controllers of nature, such as angels or deities who control different phenomena. These formless beings are human beings who have evolved and learned to control nature, and by that control earned the enjoyment of certain pleasures in the heavenly realms. But they cannot become completely liberated from these limiting desires and attachments unless they are reborn as humans and work through the desire seeds here. The coming and going will continue until all desire seeds are burned and they completely know themselves. Freedom from desire comes from clearly understanding one's nature and then letting go of attachment to the fulfillment of the desires.

Practice: Learn to observe and recognize the ego in action. Keep a watchful eye on it. When there is progress, or experiences, let go of the ensuing movement of pride coming from the ego.

20. *śraddhā-vīrya-smṛti-samādhi-prajñā-pūrvaka itareṣām*

śraddhā = faith and intense devotion

vīryam = vigour, strength, courage, dignity

smṛti = memory; mindfulness

samādhi = meditative or profound spiritual absorption

prajñā = discernment; insight, understanding

pūrvaka = previous, preceded by, attended with

itareṣam = of the others

For other [*yogins*], [the accomplishment of non-distinguished cognitive absorption] is preceded by intense devotion, courage, mindfulness, cognitive absorption and true insight.

In contrast to those *yogins* referred to in the previous verse, who leave the physical body before reaching non-distinguished cognitive absorption (*asaṁprajñātaḥ samādhi)*, those who do reach it, do so by developing the following:

śraddhā = Intense devotion with implicit faith in Yoga, with confidence in one's capacity, one's sadhana or methods, and one's preceptor;

vīryam = Energy, enthusiasm and courage arises from such faith and produces intense devotion wherein the emotions also support one's practice;

smṛti = Memory; where one remembers the path constantly, the lessons learned, so as not to fall back into a worldly perspective; one remains attentive;

samādhi = One regularly cultivates the experience of cognitive absorption. Though it is not constant due to the fluctuations of the mind *(cittavṛttiḥ)* and distractions, it develops by means of yogic *sādhana.*

prajñā = Discernment; insight. By vigilant self-awareness, moment-to-moment, one receives insights and guidance through the events of one's life.

Spiritual energy and strength brings attentiveness and vigilance. These, in turn bring recollection of one's chosen path, the discipline one is following. This memory brings continuous awareness.

Such continuous awareness brings discernment *(prajñā)* between the Real Self and the non-real.

Asaṁprajñatāh samādhi (non-object-oriented cognitive absorption) may come as an eventual consequence of the repeated experience of object-oriented cognitive absorption (*saṁprajñātaḥ samādhi)* as the subconscious tendencies gradually dissolve. However, it may also come as a result of the students cultivating certain positive tendencies, enumerated in verse I.20, such as faith, enthusiasm, vigilance, discernment and contemplation. These will create the ideal conditions by which old tendencies can be dissolved.

Practice: Cultivate faith, enthusiasm, vigilance, discernment and contemplation to dissolve the old tendencies. Repeatedly enter into distinguished cognitive absorption (*saṁprajñātaḥ samādhi)* using the *samādhi kriyās* taught during *Babaji's Kriya Yoga* level III initiation.

21. *tīvra-saṁvegānām-āsannaḥ*

tīvra-saṁvegānām = resolute
āsannaḥ = near, imminent, impending

[For those practitioners who are] utterly resolute [in their practice, the accomplishment of cognitive absorption] is imminent.

One may have glimpses of cognitive absorption *(samādhi),* the experience of the Self, in which our mind concentrates inwardly, and one is filled with absolute bliss *(ānanda),* but the real challenge is for this to become prolonged and stable. To do so one needs to practice with intense or enthusiastic devotion, to cultivate the witness consciousness and to turn the mind and senses inward, away from dispersed tendencies. When concentration and witness awareness become spontaneous and continuous, this is known as intense and resolute practice (*tīvra-saṁvega-sādhana).*

Whenever we gain a glimpse of *sadhāna* in our inner being, we would be wise to carry it into our outer life as well. It says in the *Śiva-sūtras*: "the bliss of the world is the bliss of spiritual union (*samādhi).*"

Practice: Embrace everything in the world as Divine, cultivating the universal vision of love.

22. *mṛdu-madhya-adhimātratvāt-tato' pi viśeṣaḥ*

mṛdu = mild, soft, weak

madhya = medium; moderate

adhimātratvāt = due to the intense, more than usual

tatas = from that, consequently

api = also, even, moreover

viśeṣa = characteristic difference,

Thus, the characteristic difference [as to how quickly cognitive absorption is reached depends on whether the *yogin's* practice] is weak, moderate or intense.

A mild (*mṛdhu)* practice is uneven, sporadic, full of doubts, ups and downs and full of distractions, which carry one away. A moderate (*madhya)* practice has periods of intensity and devotion, alternating with periods of forgetfulness, distractions and indulgences in negative thinking and habits. An intense practice *(adhimātra-sadhāna)* is characterized by the constant determination to remember the Self and to maintain equanimity through success, and failure, pleasure and pain, growing in love, confidence, patience and sympathy for others. It becomes intense when we worship our chosen form of God, or try to see the Divinity pervading everything, to go beyond our desires, which rise up. No matter what the intensity of the events or circumstances, no matter how great the play of the illusion *(māyā)* filled drama, we continue to see Divinity throughout.

Practice: Become immersed in doing the practices. Take a step forward every day. See everything as part of the Divine Plan, unfolding perfectly for your evolution. See nothing as outside of that Divine Plan, or contrary to it. With this in mind be persistent and consistent.

23. *īśvara-praṇidhānād-vā*

īśvara = the Lord, Siva, the Supreme Being

praṇidhānam = surrender, devotion

vā = or

Or, because of [one's] surrender to the Lord [one successfully achieves cognitive absorption]

Here Patañjali tells us that we may also achieve cognitive absorption *(samādhi)*, by surrendering our limited ego-consciousness to the Lord, or Supreme Being. He reiterates this in verse II.45. But who is the Lord? Patañjali uses the term *īśvara*. "In *Tirumantiram* verse 105, *Śiva* is described:

Beyond the two *karmas* is *Isa* seated,
The seed of this world, the mighty God become;
"This" and "That" is "*Isa*" - so the thoughtless contend,
The dross but know the basest sediment low.

For the Tamil *siddhas, Isa* is another name for the Supreme Being, *Śiva,* who is not to be confused with the limited deity with the same name in the *Vedas,* nor the one third of the trinity referred to by early Western scholars. He defies limitations or description. *Sva* means "own." Therefore, *Īśvara* means "*Śiva,* one's own Being," the Supreme Being who is immanent and transcendent in relation to all manifestation. Self-realization may come when we surrender the perspective of being apart from the Supreme Being, and recognize *Siva* as our own being. "*Jīva* becoming *Śiva*" summarizes the approach of the Tamil *yoga siddhas.* This surrender (*praṇidhāna)* must be complete, and not include any sense of some special status. It requires keen discrimination with regard to our motivations. In devotion, we feel "not my will but Thine." This perspective makes transcendence easy. As long as you feel that it is you who is doing something by your own will, you are stuck in the egoistic perspective of, "I can. I will. I can't," etc. But when we completely surrender that "I" to "Thou" we rise above nature and are free in the pure Self. This form of surrender involves feeling the existence, in the innermost core of our being, of the presence of the Lord, and to feel always that our actions are prompted by Him.

T.N. Ganapathy in his book, *The Philosophy of the Tamil Siddhas,* has given us a useful criteria: "the differentia to distinguish whether one is a *siddha,* or not, is to find out whether he or she has sung in praise of any local god or deity. In the *Tirumantiram* there is no specific reference to any local god or deity as we find in the poems of the *Āḻvārs* and the *Nāya-mārs.* The work is completely free from the lover-beloved conception of God which is the characteristic feature of the lyrical poetry of the bhakti schools." The same may be said of *Patañjali's Yoga Sūtras.***(2)** In this connection it is interesting to note that among the causes of yogic powers enumerated by Patañjali, deities do not occur.

Kailasapathy has made the relevant point that "the *siddhas* were not devotees in the sense of idol-worshippers. They believed in a supreme Abstraction. The recurrent use by the *siddhas* of the word "*civam*" in Tamil (Skt. *śiva)* is an abstract noun meaning "goodness," "auspiciousness" and the highest state of God, in which He exists as pure intelligence, in preference to the common term "*civan,*" meaning *Śiva,* makes this point very clear. In other words, they believed in an abstract idea of Godhead rather than a personal God."**(3)**

The form of God we choose, and the way we choose to express our devotion, is a matter of personal choice. However, it is easier to focus our mind upon a form, than upon something formless. Behind the countless personal forms of God, worshipped in various religions and sects, lies the Supreme Godhead.

Devotion to the Lord is not an alternative to practice and detachment in Yoga (as described in verse I.12). Patañjali shows the relationship between practice, detachment and devotion in verse II.1.

Patañjali worshipped *Śiva* at Chidambaram and at Rameswaram (where *Rāma* also worshipped *Śiva* after defeating the demon Rāvaṇa in Laṇka. There are granite statues of Patañjali at both of these *Ś*aivite shrines. In *Tirumantiram* verses 67 and 2790 it is stated that Patañjali worshipped *Śiva* at Chidambaram.

> In the splendorous temple (of Chidambaram)
> He danced,
> For the two *ṛṣis* (Patañjali and Vyagrapāda) to witness
> He danced, Form, Formless and as Cosmic Form,
> Within the Divine Grace of *Śakti.*
> He danced,
> He the *siddhas*, the *ānandas*
> As Form of Grace
> He stood and danced. (TM 2790)

Thus Self-realization is a Divine Grace, which descends upon the devotee who surrenders to the Lord. The concept of grace (*prasāda*) is found throughout the *Tirumantiram* and the writings of the other *siddhas*. How to obtain this grace? Babaji has said that winning the Grace of the Lord depends upon how much we manifest devotion for the Lord, *sādhana* (yogic practice), and service to the Lord in others. By devotion we learn what is pure love: the lover and the beloved become one. One surrenders the ego perspective. Such love brings us from duality to non-duality. By *sādhana*, which includes all forms of *Yoga* practiced to remember our Self, the subconscious is purified and duality is dissolved. We become aware of the Presence everywhere. Through service we forget our little ego-based Self and our petty problems, and we develop the universal vision of love.

Surrender to the Lord is illustrated by the story of the encounter of the divine minstrel, Nārada, with an ascetic *yogin* and a *bhakti yogin* in the forest. One day, Nārada, an angelic being, was walking through the forest. He saw a *yogin* practicing severe austerities. The *yogin* had been sitting in one spot for so many years, that the ants had built up a mound of earth over his body. He cried out when he recognized Nārada. "Oh Nārada!" he exclaimed. "I know that you are so near and dear to Lord Viṣṇu. When next you see Him, please ask him for me how much longer I must sit here before I will be allowed into his heavenly kingdom." Nārada replied, "Dear soul, certainly I will do as you request, and when next I pass through this forest, I will bring you His reply."

Nārada continued upon the path through the forest until he came to a tree where he spotted a man swinging in the branches like a monkey, chanting continuously the name of the Lord: "Rāma, Rāma!" He was a typical madcap *bhakti yogin.* When he saw Nārada, he exclaimed: "Oh, Nārada, I am so happy to see you, servant and musician of our Lord Viṣṇu. Could you please render me a service and inquire from our Lord, when I will be able to enter into His heavenly kingdom." Nārada replied, "My good soul, yes, I will be happy to inquire and I will bring you His reply the next time I pass by this way."

A few years later Nārada passed through the same forest again. When he came to the place where the ascetic *yogin* was sitting, the ascetic hailed him, exclaiming: "Oh, Nārada, how happy I am to see you. Do you have some good news for me?" Nārada replied: "Yes, and it is good news. I have spoken to Lord Viṣṇu about you and He has asked me to inform you that you will have to endure only three more births before you will enter into heaven." The ascetic replied: "What! Another three more births! I cannot wait so long!" Then he collapsed. Nārada, shook his head in compassion for the plight of the ascetic and continued on his way down the path.

When Nārada came to the tree where the madcap *bhakti yogin* was last Seen, he found him still swinging there like a monkey, chanting as usual: "Rāma, Rāma!." "Do you have some message for me from the Lord?" asked the madcap. Nārada replied: "Yes, my good fellow, but I am afraid that it is not very good news. Can you count the number of leaves in this tree? That is how many births you will have to wait before entering into heaven."

The madcap replied: "You mean I am going to enter into heaven one day! Rāma, Rāma!" he shouted with joy, and he immediately went into a divine state of ecstasy, or *samādhi.*

<u>Practice</u>: The Mother of the Sri Aurobindo Ashram recommends these ceremonial ways of cultivating surrender to the Lord, either

with a chosen image or chosen affirmations:

Three images of total surrender to the Lord:

1. to prostrate oneself at His or Her Feet in a surrender of all pride and with perfect humility;
2. to unfold our being before Him or Her, opening entirely our body from the head to the toe, as one opens a book. Spread our centers so as to make all their movements visible in a total sincerity that allows nothing to remain hidden;
3. to nestle in His or Her arms, to melt in Him with tender and absolute confidence.

Accompanied by these three affirmations:

1. May Your Will be done and not mine.
2. As You will, as You will.
3. I am Yours for Eternity.

24. *kleśa-karma-vipāka-āsayair-aparāmṛṣṭaḥ puruṣa-viśeṣa īśvaraḥ*

kleśa = affliction

karman = actions

vipāka = resultant fruit of actions

āśayair = subconscious or inner impressions, residue,

aparāmṛṣṭaḥ = untouched by

puruṣa = Self, as opposed to the "self" identified as one's per sonality or body.

viśeṣa = special

īśvara = the Lord, the Supreme Being, *Śiva*

***Ishvara* is the special Self, untouched by any afflictions, actions, fruits of actions or by any inner impressions of desires.**

The Lord, the Supreme Self, is the Self of all selves. This special Self, unlike the individual soul that is involved in nature (*prakṛti* as described in verse 17), is not affected by desires and karmic effects of desires. To realize this special Self we must let go of false identification with personality and desires. We must go beyond passing manifestations, action, desires and the afflictions of the mind. The Lord has never been under the delusion that He is in bondage to the limiting forms of nature.

Practice: Consciously let go of all of the limited identifications, definitions and description that you have about yourself. Observe yourself, your personality and your actions, and how you define your progress. Be aware how much you have grown already in the process. You may have already noticed that disturbances on the outside have less affect on you. And be aware that as the Supreme Self comes closer, your "personality" may expand, fueled with radiance from the "Sun", the higher Self. Recognize that perfection is first an inner state and not in the eye of the beholder.

25. *tatra niratiśayaṁ sarva-jña-bījam*

tatra = therein; there [in the Supreme]

niratiśaya = unsurpassed, unexcelled

sarvajñā = omniscience

bījām = source, cause, origin, seed

There [in the Supreme] the seed of the [manifestation of complete] omniscience is unsurpassed.

The Supreme Being *(īśvara)* is all knowing. All knowledge must have a source. Limited knowledge presupposes unlimited knowledge, just as all opposites have their polar opposites. The seed *(bījam)* of all knowingness exists in everything, the microcosm within the macrocosm. The seed syllable *oṁ* is such a seed of omniscience. As a seed, it is capable of growing from more to still more. By inference we may determine the existence of a Supreme Being, but not any specific information about Him.

Also see *Tirumantiram* verse 105, quoted above in the commentary on verse 23, wherein the Supreme Being is referred to as "the seed of this world."

Practice: Contemplate the meaning of *oṁ*. (See commentary on verse I.27 for the meaning)

26. *pūrveṣām-api guruḥ kālena-anavacchedāt*

pūrveṣāṁ = of the ancients, of the ancestors, of the elders

api = also

guru = teacher, spiritual parent or preceptor,

kālena = by time

anavacchedāt = unconditioned

Unconditioned by time, he is the teacher of even the most ancient teachers.

The *ṛṣis* who revealed (*śruti)* the early Hindu sacred scriptures *(the caturvedas* or the four *Vedas)*, and the *āgamas*, were inspired by the Supreme Being, *Śiva*, (and other deities) who is eternal and whose teachings are as true today as they were thousands of years ago. The absolute is not subject to changes relative to a period in history, another language or culture. Even the great *ṛṣis* and *siddhas* needed the inspiration of *Śiva* to remember what had been forgotten. In every age, the Lord makes the supreme wisdom accessible to sincere seekers. He is the idealized, eternal *yogin*, whose example inspires every generation of aspiring *yogins*. He is sometimes depicted as *Śiva* sitting atop Mount Kailash. (TM verse 20)

In *Tirumantiram* verse 67 and 68 these ancient teachers (*aṣṭanāthas* or eight *nāthas*) who were taught by *Śiva* are referred to, and Tirumūlar explains how he became one of them:

Seekest thou the Masters who *Nandi's* (*Śiva's*) grace received
First the *Nandis* four, *Śivayoga* the Holy next;
Patañjali and Vyagrapāda, who in *sabhā's* holy precincts worships
And including me to complete the number Eight. (TM 67)

By Nandi's grace I, became a spiritual master (*nāthaḥ*),
By Nandi's grace I, entered into the source (*mūlam*),
By Nandi's grace, what can I perform not?
Nandi guiding, I here below remained. (TM 68)

In a later verses 73-101 he elaborates on how he received this teaching from *Śiva* whom he personified as his spiritual teacher or *guru*, in a manner so characteristic of the Tamil *yoga siddhas*:

Our Nandi, who ever holds the bull, deer and axe
The infinite God, whose imagination is the world
Containing moving and non-moving things, has granted to me this opportunity
And on my head he planted his Holy Feet. (TM 89)

I have come by the great path of Kailash,
In the line of the Lord who expounded the above truths,
Who is eternal, Truth effulgent, limitless;
Nandi, the Blissful One who dances joyously. (TM 91)

In verse 2066, Tirumūlar says: "the Lord is the supreme guru", and in verse 2121 he adds:

The guru who admitted him into his loving Grace
Is Lord himself;
He works day by day
For the disciple's *karma* to perish
In the form of Lord
Of flowing russet locks
That wears the dripping *Gaṅgā*
The *guru* appears
And our sorrows end.

Practice: Meditate on and become absorbed in the name of the Lord, *Śiva*. Practice repetition of the mantra for *Śiva*, after receiving Initiation into it. A *mantra*, by definition, is only a *mantra* if one is initiated into it by someone who himself has been initiated and by practice absorbed into it. Follow the *mantra's* vibrations back to the source: Oneness and Bliss.

27. *tasya vācakaḥ praṇavaḥ*

tasya = its

vācakaḥ = word expressive speaking, saying, signifying

praṇava = the mystical or sacred sound *OṂ (AUM)*

The word expressive [of *īśvara*] is the mystic sound *OM* [*AUM*].

We give names to all things, all manifestation, and even the unmanifest, which is contained in it. *OṂ* is made up of three parts "A" represents creation, waking consciousness and Visnu. "U" represents preservation, dreaming, and the Supreme Spirit (*brahmā*); "M" represents destruction, dreamless sleep, and *Śiva*. "Mmm..." is beyond physical sound, is at the end, and represents *turya*, the fundamental substratum of all, the fourth level of consciousness beyond waking, dreaming and dreamless sleep. The awareness of *AUM* leads to the experience of *īśvara*, which is the Supreme Being, *Śiva*, the Absolute, containing all.

That the *siddhas* like Pataṭjali and Tirumūlar identified the supreme *mantra OṂ* with the Supreme Being, *Śiva*, or *īśvara* is indicated in *Tirumantiram* verse 953:

> When with *A*, chant *U* simultaneously
> Then does the melting (*mukti*) there appear;
> When *MA* chanted,
> With me was Nandi.
> How shall I speak of my father's greatness!

Note, the term "*mukti*" in this verse, can be translated as "absolution of the spirit from reincarnation or limiting materiality."

Practice: Chant *Oṁ* or *Oṁ kriyā babaji nāma aum* continuously for at least fifteen minutes every day in the early morning.

28. *taj-japas-tad-artha-bhāvanam*

tad = that

japas = muttering, whispering, repeating

tad = that; sometimes meaning "therefore"

artha = purpose, end and aim,

bhāvanam = feeling of devotion; contemplation

artha-bhāvanam = deliberation over a subject

[Therefore, one should] repeat [this sacred syllable *Oṁ*] while reflecting on its meaning with devotion.

Repetition of a *mantra* such as *aum* is *japaḥ*. The meaning of *aum* is given in the previous verse. *Japaḥ* purifies the mind, dissipates negative tendencies and creates a vehicle for experiencing our true essence, the Divine. As we are ruled by habits of mind, replacing such habits with *japaḥ* enables us to gain mastery over ourselves, to act consciously. Through *japaḥ*, habits lose their force and dissipate. Gradually you realize the meaning of the *mantra* as you feel it in your heart.

It must be repeated with feeling, that is, with reverence or heartfelt love for it's meaning, in order for it bring one to the Beloved. While Patañjali does not prescribe any rituals, prayers or other means of manifesting "devotion to the Lord" (*īśvara-praṇidhān*, verses I.23 and II.45) to repeat *aum* with feeling and reflection upon its meaning, is consistent with the Tamil *siddha* emphasis on internal worship, rather than temple worship.

By repeatedly chanting *Oṁ (Aum)* the mind becomes one-pointed in concentration, leading to distinguished cogntive absorption (*saṁprajñātaḥ samādhi)*, and from that ultimately non-distinguished cognitive absorption *(asaṁprajñātaḥ samādhi)* is achieved.

The effect of repeatedly chanting a *mantra* like *Oṁ* or its variant, *Aum*, is not unlike what happens to us when we listen to classical music with stereo headphones: "we" disappear; that is, "who we think we are," our thoughts, cease to exist, and what remains, is only the music, and of course pure consciousness, the Seer.

Sri Aurobindo said that when *Oṁ* is chanted correctly, with aspiration, not mechanically, it might very well help the openings upward, as well as the descent of the Divinity.

Practice: Chant *Oṁ* remembering the Supreme Lord, with joy, elation, warmth of enthusiasm, aspiration, as if you are touching His Feet, or His heart, with each sound.

29. *tataḥ pratyakcetanā-adhigamo' py-antarāya-abhāvaś-ca*

tataḥ = from this

pratyak-cetanā = inner Self awareness, one whose thoughts are turned inwards;

adhigamaḥ = attainment

api = also

antarāya = obstacle

abhāvaḥ = disappearance

ca = and

[From this practice] comes the attainment of the "inner Self awareness" and the disappearance of [all] obstacles.

When our consciousness flows towards outer sensations we identify with our reactions to these sensations. By following the sound of "Aum" inwardly to it's source, we get beyond the surface waves and begin to experience our Universal Self. Substitute the sound of "Aum" for the thoughts, and dissolve the ego glue, which causes identification with fluctuations arising within consciousness. Both the *Vedas* and tantric teachings extol the use of mantras for the purpose of Self-realization. Meditation on "Aum" is known as *oṁkāra dhyāna* and has a privileged position in *Babaji's Kriya Yoga*. As inward attention develops it turns the flow of consciousness towards the inner, true Self. The chanting must be done repeatedly and for extended periods of time.

The sound or thought of the *mantra* replaces the "I" thought as one practices *japaḥ*. As the "I" thought disappears, the obstacles (which are listed in the next verse) including sensuality, doubt, disease, etc., have nothing to hang onto. One ceases to feed the trivial round of habitual thoughts, and so they lose their force gradually and dissipate. Calm Self-awareness remains. This is the beauty of *japaḥ*. One does not have to struggle with desires and fears. One simply redirects one's mental energy away from them by concentrating on the *mantra*. Gradually they wither. Desires and fears are like cats: if one feeds them, they multiply. If one stops feeding them, they go elsewhere.

Practice: Chant often, and always with a feeling of reverence, particularly when there are strong desires or anxieties. Afterwards become quiet and meditate on "*Aum*."

30. *vyādhi-styāna-saṁśaya-pramāda-ālasya-avirati-bhrānti-darśana-alabdha-bhūmikatva-anavasthitatvāni citta-vikṣepās-te'ntarāyāḥ*

vyādhi = disease, ailment

styāna = dullness, rigidity

saṁśaya = doubt, hesitation

pramāda = carelessness, negligence

ālasya = laziness, idleness

avirati = lack of detachment, sense indulgence,

bhrānti = false, confusing, wrong

darśana = view, observation, understanding
alabdha = failure, unobtained

bhūmikatva = "firm ground", stage, place, basis

anavasthitatvāni = instability,

citta = consciousness

vikṣepāḥ = distractions, dispersion

te = these

antarāyāḥ = obstacles

Disease, dullness, doubt, carelessness, laziness, sense indulgence, false perception, failure to reach firm ground and instability - these distractions of consciousness are obstacles.

The obstacles to inner awareness, or witnessing, are the nine distractions listed here. However they are not insurmountable. Through the practice of surrender to the Lord *(īśvara-praṇidhānaḥ)*, as described above, including *japaḥ* with devotion, as well as the cultivation of their opposites, and other yogic *sadhānas*, including selfless service to others *(karma yoga)*, they may be overcome.

Disease *(vyādhi)* is both physical and mental. It results from how we react to the stress of life.

Dullness (*styāna)* occurs when there is not adequate energy we cannot keep a continuous awareness. We must not waste energy and must avoid fatigue.

Doubt *(saṁśaya)* is the tendency of the mind to question, and when it is not accompanied by a seeking for answers, it may leave one cynical and unprepared to continue to make efforts.

Carelessness *(pramāda)* is inattention, dispersion, and a habitual lack of focus.

Laziness (*ālasya) is* a habit, due to discouragement, lack of enthusiasm or inspiration.
Sense indulgence or sense addiction (*avirati)* occurs where desires are not detached from, but rather encouraged.

False perception (*bhrānti)* is not seeing the underlying reality.

Failure to reach firm ground (*alabdha bhūmikatva)* occurs when there is lack of patience and perseverance.

Instability (*anavasthitatva)* is the failure to maintain equilibrium during the highs and lows of life due to a lack of consistency in one's practice; getting lost in the transitory show.

Practice: Make a list of how the above obstacles show up in your life. Be specific as to which ones affect you the most in order of importance. Cultivate their opposites using techniques of autosuggestion and affirmation. Start with the ones which affect you the least, clear them up, and travel up the list. (See reference **4** for assistance with auto-suggestions).

31. *duḥkha-daurmanasya-aṅgam-ejayatva-śvāsa-praśvāsā vikṣepa-sahabhuvaḥ*

duḥkha = anxiety, pain, difficulty

daurmanasya = depression, despair

aṅga = body, limb

ejayatva = trembling, shaking, unsteady

śvāsa = inhalation, breathing

praśvāsa = exhalation

vikṣepaḥ = distraction

sahabhuvaḥ = accompanying, appearing together

The accompaniments of [these] distractions are trembling in the body, unsteady inhalation, [of the breath] depression and anxiety. The mental distractions *(vikṣepāḥ)* are those movements, which cause us to forget, or lose, inner awareness. When we become very absorbed by our thoughts, and lose our equilibrium, there may even be side effects in our emotions, like depression (*daurmanasya)*, anxiety *(duḥkha)*, trembling in the physical body, or absence of calm, even breathing (*ejayatva-śvāsa-praśvāsā)*. Such movements which accompany these mental distractions may serve to remind us just how much we have lost sight of our true Self and thus help us to return to it. We can chant or do loving actions to change our emotions, or breathe deeply, or do postures to quiet the mind, emotions and body. Psychological treatments are generally palliative and symptomatic, but such yogic activities go to the real causal part of our nature. The body-mind has a will and a memory of its own, which was well-known in ancient times. A wholistic approach such as *Yoga* will prevent such accompaniments from creating major illnesses.

Practice: When troubled or confused, do *yoga āsanas*. Clarity will come. Or sit quietly in an *āsana* and just breathe with awareness. Practice conscious breathing, to the point that this slow, deep, smooth breathing becomes natural, all of the time.

32. *tat-pratiṣedha-artham-eka-tattva-abhyāsaḥ*

tad = that (referring here to *artha*)

pratiṣedha = preventing, keeping back

artham = purpose, meaning

eka = single

tattvam = subject, principle, literally translated as "thatness"

abhyāsaḥ = consistent, repeated practice,

The practice of concentration on a single subject is the best way to prevent [the obstacles and their accompaniments].

The practice of concentration on a single subject (*eka-tattva-abhyāsaḥ)* keeps the mind from getting dispersed, or lost in its thoughts. Inner awareness grows. The obstacles, such as dullness *(styāna)*, sickness *(vyādhi)*, laziness (*ālasya)*, doubt *(saṁśaya)*, carelessness *(pramāda)* and sensual indulgence (*avirati),* and their accompaniments, such as anxiety *(duḥkha)* and depression (*daurmanasya),* gradually retreat. All of the *yogas* involve concentration on a subject: the body (*aṅga),* the breathing, a *mantra,* meditation (*dhyāna).*

By using the object as a symbol, we can develop clarity and steadiness of vision, which in turn will permit us to ultimately transcend the subject and realize our true Being. The subjects will vary according to taste, but the goal, Self realization, is the same.

The tendency of the mind to get dispersed keeps us stuck in the illusion of separateness: one fails to experience union with the All. Thoughts often repeated give rise to the illusion of permanence and invite the invasion of unwanted visitors: the obstacles and their accompaniments.

The word "*tattvam*" also refers to the twenty-four principles found in *prakriti* according to the philosophical system of *Sāṅkhya yoga,* and to the ninety-six enumerated principles of nature in *Tirumantiram* verses 125, 154, and 381-410. The Tamil *siddhas* were first-rate scientists, who studied Nature, in all of its forms, and at all levels. Rather than seeking to simply transcend Nature, or go beyond the world of manifestation, they studied it and organized their understanding of it in the system of the *tattvas.* By appreciating Nature, in all of its manifestations, they were able to realize the Supreme Being.

The term *tattuvam* in Tamil is composed of two parts: "*tat*" which means "It," ie. "*civam*" (Skt. *Śiva),* "*tuvam*" (the suffix û*tva* in Sanskrit) means It's nature. To know the true nature of the human soul and of the Supreme is the philosophy of "tattuvam."**(5)**

It is generally easier to concentrate on a form than on something without form, therefore in the early stages of developing one-pointedness, the choice of an object with form is recommended. If it is an object which one finds fascinating or uplifting, it will be easier, as the mind will be less inclined to wander. Ultimately, one may concentrate on *Īśvara* itself or on the sense of "I."

Practice: Focus your attention on a single object, such as a candle flame, with eyes open, or in meditation, with eyes closed, visualize a single object, or follow the breath or repeat a *mantra.* Concentrate regularly on the form of your chosen deity (your *ista devatā).* For example the form of *Babaji, Kṛṣṇa, Śiva* or the Divine Mother, not only during meditation, but throughout the day. Choose one that you are attracted to, that resonates with you. Allow your chosen deity to come close to you, to be with you when you worship, to come alive through your picture or image. Be aware of the Divine Presence walking with you, speaking with you, guiding you and carrying you when necessary. Laugh with the Divine (Babaji's Kriya Yoga level III initiation).

33. *maitrī-karuṇā-muditā-upekṣāṇāṁ sukha-duḥkha-puṇya-apuṇya-viṣayāṇāṁ bhāvanātaś-citta-prasādanam*

maitrī = friendship, goodwill

karuṇā = compassion

muditā = delight, rejoicing

upekṣānāṁ = equanimity

sukha = happy, pleasure

duḥkha = unhappy, dissatisfaction, suffering, anxiety

puṇya = virtuous; meritorious,

apuṇya = wicked; non-virtuous, lacking merit

viṣayāṇāṁ = of conditions, of objects

bhāvanātaḥ = from cultivation, producing

citta = consciousness

prasādanam = undisturbed calmness, tranquility,

By cultivating attitudes of friendship towards the happy, compassion for the unhappy, delight in the virtuous and equanimity towards the non-virtuous, the consciousness retains its undisturbed calmness.

The mind can be an obstacle or an aid in the process of Self-realization. To facilitate it, the cultivation of these four attitudes is recommended in daily life. Even if we do not aspire toward spiritual goals, following this advice will make anyone's life serene. The mind has a tendency to do the opposite at times.

Friendship or goodwill (*mettā*) towards the happy (*sukha*): It is necessary to cultivate this because we sometimes feel jealous or envious toward those who are happy and are censorious toward them. For example, if someone is enjoying the fruits of their labor in a material way, we may be jealous. Rather we should say: "May they continue to prosper time and again."

Compassion (*karuṇā*) towards those who are suffering (*duḥkha*): Even if what we can do by our thoughts or our actions for another is only a little, by opening ourselves to the compassion, our own mind and emotions are transformed. We should avoid judging them by saying, for example, "they suffer because of their bad *karma*."

Delight (*muditā*) in the virtuous (*puṇya*): Emulate them and rejoice that such persons exist.

Equanimity (*upekṣā*) towards the non-virtuous (*apuṇya*): Do not allow the mind to be colored by such negative persons. Do not judge others. Nor should we disregard those who may be suffering, but love them as well. We may love someone, without judging their behavior. Judging others only reinforces in our own minds the negative qualities we are condemning. We generally condemn in others what we harbor in ourselves. The world is within us. To change the world, we can change our thoughts. Overlook the lapses of others. Do not dwell on their weaknesses. By dwelling on their weaknesses we transmit thoughts to them which only reinforce their weaknesses.

By cultivating these attitudes, the mind becomes purified, and one-pointed serenity results.

Practice: Meditate on, and cultivate friendliness towards the happy, compassion for the unhappy, delight in the virtuous, and equanimity towards the non-virtuous. Use interpersonal relations to develop these qualities, and be aware of ensuing calmness.

34. *pracchardana-vidhāraṇābhyāṁ vā prāṇasya*

pracchardana = exhalation
vidhāraṇābhyāṁ = of the retention of

vā = or

prāṇasya = of the breath; of life

Or [that undisturbed calmness of consciousness is achieved] by the [careful] exhalation and the retention of the breath.

By refining the breath *(prāṇa)* through breath awareness and slow even four part breathing with ratios such as 1:0:2:0 or 2:0:2:0, the senses and mind become calm. The figures refer to the relative lengths of the inhalation, interval between inhalation and exhalation, exhalation, and finally, the interval between the exhalation and the next inhalation. The zero indicates avoidance of holding the breath. By watching the breath come slowly in and out, equilibrium is created. The mind and breath are closely connected; every psychological state has a corresponding breathing pattern. When the breath slows, the mental activity also slows. When the mind gets agitated, so does the breath. So we can get control of the mind by controlling the breath. This verse is not about breath control *(prāṇāyāma)*, but breath awareness with slow, even breathing, hence the special term used. It is suggestive of the practice of the "*haṁsaḥ*" meditation as well as the "walking meditation with coordinated breathing," familiar to students of *Babaji's Kriya Yoga*.

In Tirumantiram verse 567 we find:

> "Let *prāṇa* merge in Mind,
> And together the two be stilled
> Then no more shall birth and death be
> Therefore learn to direct breath."

In the space between the inhalation and the exhalation, Truth may easily be perceived.

Breath awareness may be practiced anytime and for extended periods, and it particularly applicable when the mind is unsettled. Through it, cognitive absorption (*samādhi)* may be realized.

Practice: "*Hamsaḥ*" meditation; also the "walking meditation" with coordinated breathing taught in *Babaji's Kriya Yoga*.

35. *viṣaya-vatī vā pravṛttir-utpannā manasaḥ sthiti-nibandhanī*

viṣayavatī = taking upon oneself an object of the senses,

vā = or

pravṛttiḥ = activity, moving onward; cognition

utpannā = brought about, arisen, born, produced

manasaḥ = of the mind

sthitiḥ = steadiness

nibandhanī = holding, binding, causing

Or the holding of the mind steady is brought about by cognitive [focus within] the field of the senses.

The subtle senses are the focus of attention in several of *Babaji's Kriya Yoga dhyānas and kriyās,* or meditation techniques. In the dream (*svapna)* state they are experienced without attention. By making their experience the subject of meditation, one stands back from mental agitation and directs the flow of thoughts. Calmness (*prasādanam*) and steadiness (*sthitiḥ)* develop. They can also be experienced as clairvoyance, clairsentience, for example, viewing one's aura around the nose, or fingertips, or around another person. When the mind is dispersed, there is no awareness, and therefore no calmness.

Concentration on the tip of the nose gives higher smell perception. Concentration on the tip of the tongue gives super-sensuous taste, that on the tongue, super-sensuous touch and that at the root of the tongue, super-sensuous sound, according to Swami Hariharananda Aranya.

Practice: Practice the visualization or concentration exercises involving any of the five subtle senses.

36. *viśokā vā jyotiṣmatī*

viśoka = blissful, sorrowless

vā = or

jyotiṣmatī = from *jyotis*: supreme light, illumination; + *matī*: having, possessing

Or [by concentrating on the] ever blissful supreme light within [one leaves behind all suffering and one experiences lucidity].

Another way to calm the mind is to imagine a bright light or a candle flame inside of ourselves, for example, in the forehead, heart, or any of the *cakras*. Eventually, we will experience the Reality of the Presence of the Divine Light everywhere. Many traditions talk about the experience of the Divine Light - *jyoti*, or "Vision of the Golden Light." In *Kriya Yoga*, there are several *dhyāna kriyās* which involve this vision, "the Three Divine Qualities, as well as Concentration or *trāṭaka* on a candle. This permits subconscious impressions (*saṁskāras)* to subside and we experience ourselves as a vast ocean of light. Calmness comes, because one goes beyond the level of duality where there is a diversity of thoughts, to the Absolute plane, where all is perceived as light like the ocean. Lucidity occurs when the sediment settles. Light permeates everything, but we rarely notice it because we are preoccupied with the forms. Like the images in a film, we miss the screen, the presence. Christ said: "I am the Light."

One way to practice this is to imagine in one's heart a limitless, sky-like or transparent effulgence; then think that the self is within that, i.e. "I am spread all over it."

Practice: Practice the *sārūpya jyoti samādhi dhyāna kriyā* taught in *Babaji's Kriya Yoga* level III initiation.

37. *vīta-rāga-viṣayaṁ vā cittam*

vīta = free, released, gone away

rāga = attachment, passion

viṣayaṁ = object
vā = or

citta = consciousness

Or [that undisturbed calmness of mind is achieved when] consciousness [is directed towards the minds of those great souls] who have conquered attachment.

In the previous verses Patañjali mentions obstacles, and accompaniments, which disturb the mind, as well as various means to calm them. In this verse we learn that calmness can be cultivated in the mind by concentrating on the mind of one who has become pure, "a great soul." Such a person has freed him or herself from all desire, fear, anger and greed, which disturb the mind. Their vibrations and nature soothe our troubled mind and by the principle of sympathetic vibrations we also grow calm and free from attachment. This permits their being, mind and energy to direct our own, and we become their instrument, no longer under the illusion of being a separate doer.

This practice is referred to in *Tirumantiram* and is also current in *Babaji's Kriya Yoga.*

Practice: Meditate upon great spiritual personalities. Allow their qualities to be absorbed within you.

38. *svapna-nidrā-jñāna-ālambanaṁ vā*

svapna = dream

nidrā = sleep

jñāna = knowledge, consciousness, wisdom

ālambana = base, supporting, receptacle, abode

vā = or

Or [that undisturbed calmness of mind] is supported by the knowledge that arises in dreams and sleep.

The mind may remember it's serenity and calm state by recalling dreams, which brought it to a higher state, or by recalling the peace it felt during deep sleep. It is not the sleepiness one should recall, but the peace. In special visionary dreams we experience higher being,

Divine Light, and new states of well being. The memory of this may inspire us to return to our true Self whose nature is Being, Consciousness, Bliss.

As our inner consciousness grows with our *sadhāna*, these visionary dreams may increase in number and clarity. Greater understanding will come.

Practice: Keep a record of dreams in a diary. Dreams may be used as objects of contemplation.

39. *yathā-abhimata-dhyānād-vā*

yathā = as

abhimata = desired

dhyānād = from meditation or contemplation

vā = or

Or from the subject of meditation [choosing anything] as desired

We may choose any object we like, but it should ideally be something that is fascinating and uplifting. He has already mentioned many objects in the previous verses. The mind is drawn to various sense objects, or subjects, according to the person's interests and desires. By allowing ourselves to focus on what we desire, the mind can explore and find its limits. Gradually our interests will evolve from external things, to things seen internally only, like *cakras, nāḍis,* deities, light, metaphysical concepts. By focusing on them the mind turns away from dispersion and finds calm and one-pointedness, in preparation for *samādhi.*

Practice: Choose one subject and stay with that subject. Practice the second *dhyāna kriyā.*

40. *parama-aṇu-parama-mahat(t)va-anto' sya vaśīkāraḥ*

parama = most, extreme, limit primal atom

aṇu = small, fine, minute

parama = most

maha(t)tva = greatness, size, extent, magnitude

antaḥ = end, conclusion

asya = his, of him

vaśīkāraḥ = mastery

[Gradually one's] mastery [of concentration] extends from the most minute [primal atom] to the greatest magnitude.

Yogins are able to hold their minds steady in relation to any object, from the smallest subatomic particle, to the entire universe. Everything becomes accessible to such persons. Having gained mastery over the mind nothing is difficult to meditate upon.

One develops the *siddhis* of lightness (*laghiman)* and (*mahiman*), awareness of the micro and macrocosm; by focusing the usually dispersed mind on an object (*saṁyama* or communion), one becomes it and can manifest it - power of materialization, and all of the siddhis, or yogic miraculous powers, develop. So from steadiness of mind all these divine powers can develop.

Practice: Meditate upon objects in nature from those at the subatomic level, through the visible, invisible and cosmic levels.

41. *kṣīṇa-vṛtter-abhijātasya-iva maṇer-grahītṛ-grahaṇa-grāhyeṣu tat-stha-tad-añjanatā samāpattiḥ*

kṣīṇa = dwindled or weakened , diminished

vṛttiḥ = fluctuations
abhijāta = precious, noble

iva = like

maṇes = of a gem or jewel

grahītṛ = knower, grasper

grahaṇa = knowing, grasping

grāhyeṣu = known, in the grasped

tad = that, it

stha = standing, staying abiding

tad = that it

añjanatā = assuming the color of any object

samāpattiḥ = cognitive absorption with identification with the object of contemplation; coincidence; unity; coming together

Just as a pure crystal assumes the colors [or shapes] of objects standing nearby, so cognitive absorption [occurs] when the fluctuations [of consciousness], having dwindled [by various means], knower, known and their relationship becomes indistinguishable.

Here the process of attaining *samādhi* is described. When the fluctuations of consciousness (*cittavṛttiḥ)* including perceptions through the senses, conceptualizations, memories, etc. see vs. I.2 and I.5) have dwindled, due to the various practices described in previous verses, the *yogin* no longer sees the difference between himself, objects of knowledge and knowing itself (or the meditator, meditated upon and meditation). When the difference between subject and object disappears, the process of knowing also disappears. The mind becomes completely absorbed and takes the form of it's object of meditation like a clear crystal, which reflects the form of a flower placed near to it. When the mind is absorbed in the thought of a saint or other great soul, it will reflect the qualities of such a saint. The mind will therefore reflect what it becomes absorbed by.

Practice: Meditate with the guru seated in the center of your heart shining like a pure crystal. Become absorbed in That, I AM.

42. *tatra śabda-artha-jñāna-vikalpaiḥ saṁkīrṇa savitarkā samāpattiḥ*

tatra = wherein, there, in that

śabda = sound, word

artha = object, meaning, purpose

jñāna = knowledge

vikalpaiḥ = by or with imagination, conceptualization

saṁkīrṇā = mixed, interspersed; indistinct

savitarkā = with observation, thought, reasoning, reflection

samāpattiḥ = cognitive absorption wherein one identifies with the object of contemplation; coincidence

The cognitive absorption wherein subject-object identification is mixed with spontaneous words, objects and knowledge about material objects, is known as "*savitarkā samadhi*": *Samadhi* with reflection.

In this verse and the following two verses I.43-44, Patanjali analyzes "*saṁprajñāta samādhi*," referred to as "distinguished" or "object-oriented" cognitive absorption (see verse I.17). He distinguishes four gradations in it: "*savitarkā*" ("departing from a material object with reflection"), "*nirvitarkā*" ("departing from a material object without reflection"), "*savicāra*" ("departing from a subtle object with reflection") and "*nirvicāra*" ("departing from a subtle object without reflection"). During the first level of cognitive absorption (*samādhi)*, referred to as *savitarkā* (from '*sa*' meaning 'with', '*vi*' meaning 'to and fro' and '*tarkā*' meaning 'reflection'), identification between oneself and the material, visible object of meditation may be interspersed with supra-cognitive insights and conceptualizations about the material or visible object of meditation. They arise spontaneously. The visible or material object might be the form of a saint, a yantra, anything from nature. Such things are often taken as the object of meditation exercises.

These are not the result of wandering thoughts, or vague ideas, as in ordinary thinking. The clarity and force of the insight is unique. The fact that they can arise at all indicates the incomplete degree of subject-object absorption (*samādhi*) achieved. Also the words, objects and insights may arise independently and separate from one another, between periods of absorption (*samādhi).*

Practice: While meditating upon a visualized form, or with eyes open on a visible material object, such as a candle flame or the *Śiva lingaṁ* stone, allow insights to arise spontaneously and effortlessly, in between the inhalation and exhalation. Learn and practice the *dhyāna kriyās,* taught in *Babaji's Kriya Yoga* level I initiation.

43. *smṛti-pariśuddhau sva-rūpa-śūnya-iva-artha-mātra-nirbhāsā nirvitarkā*

smṛti = impressions, memories

pariśuddhau = purified or clean

svarūpa = own-form

śūny = empty

iva = as it were, like, as if, "seems to be"

artha = object, form

mātra = only

nirbhāsā = shines forth, is illumined

nirvitarkā = without reflection

The cognitive absorption wherein subject-object identification is well purified of impressions, and one has become, as it were, empty, in one's own form only, shining without reflection is "*nirvitarkā samādhi.*"

Absorption without the accompaniment of thought *(nirvitarkā samādhi)* occurs when there is a complete cessation of supra-cognitive insights and conceptualizations regarding the material, or visible, objects of meditation. Unlike absorption accompanied by thought (*savitarkā samādhi* in verse I.42) the subject-object identification is complete. No more supra-cognitive insights arise between periods of absorption on the visible or material object of meditation. The knower is known.

Practice: While meditating on visualized form, or with eyes open on a material visible object such a *Śiva lingaṁ* stone, allow the space between the breaths to expand and allow all thoughts to subside into Stillness.

44. *etayā-eva savicārā nirvicārā ca sūkṣma-viṣayā vyākhyātā*

etayā = in the same way

eva = thus

savicāra = reflective; with subtle reflection

nirvicāra = super or non-reflective; without subtle reflection

ca = and

sūkṣma = subtle, fine

viṣayā = objects (see vs. I.11), condition

vyākhyātā = explained, fully detailed

Similarly explained are the [states of cognitive absorption wherein the subject-object identification] is mixed with words and reflections about subtle objects, "*savicara*" [*samadhi*] and without words and reflections, "*nirvicara*" [*samadhi*].

With reference to verse I.17, subtle objects are abstractions without reference to material observation. For example, such abstractions may be "Love", "Purity", "Bliss", "Being", "God." They may be themselves the objects of exercises in the first stages of training the mind to meditate. As in verse I.42 the spontaneous insights or conceptualizations arise from a supra-cognitive source as flashes of inspiration, not as vague mental wanderings. This is known as "*savicāra samādhi*."

As in verse I.43 when we cease to identify with such abstractions (see verse I.2), that is, the mind is empty and only the feeling of "I am" remains, with no more mixture of ideas or reflections about abstractions, it is "*nirvicāra* (non-reflective) *samādhi*."

Practice: While meditating upon abstractions or concepts, during the space between the inhalation and exhalation, allow insights to arise spontaneously and effortlessly. Learn and practice *arūpya dhyāna kriyā* in *Babaji's Kriya Yoga* level I initiation. Later allow the space between the breaths to expand and allow all thoughts to subside into Stillness.

45. *sūkṣma-viṣayatvaṁ ca-aliṅga-paryavasānam*

sūkṣma = subtle

viṣayatva = objectness, nature of a condition

ca = and

aliṅga = unmanifest; according to Vyasa, *prakriti,* the most subtle cause

paryavasānam = including, end, termination

The subtle nature of objects terminate in the unmanifest.

In verse I.45 Patanjali describes how the repeated experience of non-reflective cognitive absorption, whether supported by a material or subtle object as a point of departure, ultimately leads to a continuous state of cognitive of absorption known as "*asaṁprajñāta samādhi*." The experience of the mind, first with material or visible objects of nature, then with the subtler objects, such as abstractions, dissolves in the ultimate Source: the most subtle cause. This is the realm of the transcendental, core reality beyond which the "*buddhiḥ*" or intellect can grasp. One cannot measure the ocean with a teacup, nor can one measure the ultimate reality with our discriminative faculty. This is why "those who know *samādhi* do not talk about, and those who do not know *samādhi* talk about it." In Self-realization, there is no more distinction between the knower, the known, and knowing. Silence rules. The Seer remains.

Practice: While meditating upon abstractions or concepts, allow the space between the breaths to expand and allow all thoughts to subside into Stillness.

46. *tā eva sabījaḥ samādhiḥ*

tāh = these

eva = indeed (emphatic)

sabīja = with seed; with primary cause

samādhi = cognitive absorption

These very cognitive absorptions possess seed [s].

One may wonder at this point: "What kind of life is possible after such an experience?" *Yogins* often fall into the trap of assuming that because they have experienced *samādhi* of one type or another, that they are automatically a saint, or have reached the highest stage of perfection. It should be emphasized that *samādhi* is a mental state, in which the mind becomes for the most part, silent. The four types of *samādhi* mentioned in verses I.42-I.44 and I.47 "*savitarkā*," "*nirvitarkā*," "*nirvicāra*," and "*nirvicāra*," are all threatened by the existence of seed-like latent cognitive afflictions. These lie in the subconscious mind awaiting the right circumstances to sprout. Until they have been burnt by the fire of *sādhana* and in the highest form of *samādhi*, there is always the risk that the *yogin*'s consciousness will again assume the forms arising from the subconscious and that Self-awareness will be replaced by ego-identification (see verse I.4). The *yogin* may find himself in a kind of elevator, going "up" into *samādhi* during periods of intense practice and going down into the field of mental distraction and neuroses at other times. This "up and down elevator" syndrome is recalled in verse IV.27: "In between, distracting thoughts may arise due to past impressions." This explains why so many *yogins* adept at going into states of *samādhi,* are just as neurotic as the next person when they come down. Even worse, they may use their "experience" of *samādhi* to enlarge their ego, or to justify abusive behavior towards others, or even to stop their yogic discipline. One should beware of *yogins* who seek to justify immoral behavior because of their so-called spiritual experiences.

The remedy to falling into such a trap of spiritual pride is given in verse IV.28, wherein Patanjali reminds us of how to remove the causes of afflictions, given in verses II.1, 2, 10, 11 and 26, using intense practice and detachment.

Practice: Use every moment, every event, to "let go" of what disturbs the peace in the mind. Release reactions. Cultivate contentment. Be equal minded in the face of the dualities of life. (But carefully and consciously look at whatever seeds sprout as well, until they do no more.)

47. *nirvicāra-vaiśāradye' dhyātma-prasādaḥ*

nirvicāra = super-reflective or non-reflective; beyond reflection

vaiśāradye = lucid, clearness of intellect

*adhyātma*n = supreme Self

prasādaḥ = undisturbed calmness

In the pristine state of *nirvicāra samādhi* [absorption without words and reflection] the supreme Self [shines] in undisturbed calmness.

Undisturbed by any movement pertaining even to the subtlest of objects, the *yogin* remains in a heightened awareness, identified with the supreme Self, pure, clear and shining. Only the feeling "I am" remains. One has gone beyond a passing experience to a continuous, permanent state of Being. One has passed from the experience of Self-realization or Enlightenment, to the permanent state of Self-realization or Enlightenment.

It is significant that Patañjali uses the term undisturbed calmness (*prasādaḥ*, see verse I.33). In such a state of calmness, the myriad manifestations of nature do not disturb the fundamental realization of "I am." One remains in the world but not of it. Stillness is a further step beyond calmness, wherein there is no awareness of anything but that undifferentiated being. Calmness is not the absence of thoughts or emotions, but being present with them.

Practice: Practice being actively calm and calmly active. Be present in all activities and throughout all the reactions of the mind. Practice the technique of continual bliss (*nityānanda kriyā)* as taught in *Babaji's Kriya Yoga* level II initiation.

48. *ṛtaṁ-bharā tatra prajñā*

ṛtaṁ = truth, *dharma,* order

bharā = bearing, carrying

tatra = there

prajñā = wisdom, knowledge, intelligence; literally onward (*pra)* + to know *(jñā);* awareness

In that [*nirvicāra samādhi*] [state of absorption without words and reflection] awareness is truth bearing.

In ordinary physical consciousness, knowledge *(prajñā)* is acquired through the senses, or by reasoning. But in *samādhi* it comes by direct cognition or insight and is "truth-bearing," meaning without error. One knows by intuitive perception the truth of things directly by becoming one with them. A sixth sense or psychic knowing permits this. By identity with the manifestations of nature (*prakṛti*), the *yogin* becomes a sage and can express himself or herself accurately on any subject even though not educated in it. What Georg Feuerstein has termed "the vision of discernment"(6) is further described by Patañjali in verses II.26 and III.49.

Practice: Notice the insights and wisdom, which arise in such states. They are original and make one feel good (connected) in a striking manner.

49. *śruta-anumāna-prajñābhyām-anya-viṣayā viśeṣa-arthatvāt*

śruta = that which is heard from tradition or scripture

anumāna = inference

prajñābhyām = from the knowledge

anya = distinct

viṣayā viśeṣa = this special truth

arthatvāt = purpose

This special truth has a distinct purpose apart from knowledge, inference, or scriptural study.

Here Patanjali distinguishes these "truth bearing insights" arising in "*nirvicāra samādhi*" from the words, knowledge and reflections described in I.42. When we acquire this "truth bearing" insight (*ṛtaṁ-bhāra prajñā)* we transcend the mind and can therefore realize the Supreme Being and the Self. No orally transmitted teachings (*śruti)* or logical inference (*anumāna)* can reveal the truth of the Supreme Being or the Self, because the mind cannot grasp anything more subtle than itself. One may compare such inner-realizations with their descriptions in sacred scriptures or with one's own inferences, by reasoning, but even this is not necessary. Self-realization occurs when the mind becomes silent. As the Psalmist said: "Be Still and Know that I am God."

Practice: Be aware and acknowledge with love and gratitude how often you are in a state of grace.

50. *taj-jaḥ saṁskāro' nya-saṁskāra-pratibandhī*

tad = that

jaḥ = born, arisen, sprung from , produced from

saṁskāra = subconscious impression

anya = other

pratibandhī = obstructing, preventing, impeding

The subconscious impressions produced from that [truth bearing awareness] will impede [the arising of any] other subconscious impressions.

The pure, non-reflective, state of cognitive insight effectively restrains the externalization of consciousness into old forms, thoughts or habits. The *yogin* will not be attached to anything. The background has become the foreground in the *yogin*'s field of consciousness - the feeling of "I am" rules. While the *yogin* may continue to live a normal life, it is without attachment to anything, except the impression of "I am." As Aurobindo put it succinctly (and quite humorously): "I have lost the habit of thinking." When this state is achieved, all will be accomplished by a higher consciousness. The *yogin* is no longer on the "up and down elevator" between neurosis and the "experience" of Self-realization. The *yogin* is enlightened: a state of effortless and continual Self-realization, or effulgent awareness, is present at all times.

Practice: Self-realization is now effortless and continual. Allow the old habits of thinking to be replaced by this new higher consciousness and movement. Be That, and allow it to work through you.

51. *tasya-api nirodhe sarva-nirodhān-nirbījaḥ samādhiḥ*

tasya-api = even of this

nirodhe = with the cessation; see I.2
sarva = all

nirodhān = having ceased or having been restrained

nirbījaḥ = seedless

samādhiḥ = cognitive absorption

With the cessation [of identifying with] even this last impression, ["I am,"] all [others] having been restrained, there results the seedless "*nirbija*" cognitive *samadhi.*

Like the proverbial stick, which is used to poke the fire and is at last itself cast into the fire, even the last impression "I am, " used to detach the Self from identification with objects (*prakriti*) of consciousness, is detached from. What remains is effulgent Self awareness, independent of all. There is no more division between the knower and the known, not even the feeling of "I have realized God," no more birth nor death.

Tirumūlar defines *samadhi* or Self-knowledge as a state where the "I" becomes or is the "He":

> He and he know Him not;
> If he knows Him, then Knower is he not;
> If he knows Him
> Then he the Knower and He the Known
> Become but one. (TM 1789)

Practice: Reflect on this: "Are you willing and ready for a state where you will want to have nothing; a state where you will know nothing; a state where you will be no one at all?"

Chapter 2: SĀDHANA-PĀDA

"*Sādhana*" means "discipline." The Tamil *yoga siddhas* have a famous saying: "The amount of happiness in life is proportional to one's discipline." It includes all that we may do to remember the truth of our being, and to let go of what we are not. In this chapter, Patañjali prescribes *kriyā yoga* as the *sādhana* or "path to Self-realization." Feuerstein has pointed out that the verses related to *aṣṭāṅga yoga* ("the eight-fold Yoga") appear to be quoted in the text of Patañjali.(1) Patañjali's *kriyā yoga*, as indicated in verse II.1 and as discussed in the introduction involves intense practice (*tapas)*, detachment (*vairāgya)*, self-study (*svādhyāya*) and devotion to the Lord (*īśvara-praṇidhāna)*. But as few are prepared for this, Patañjali appears to have recommended *aṣṭāṅga yoga* as preliminary practices. It is indeed ironic that Patañjali's name is associated today with *aṣṭāṅga yoga* rather that with *kriyā yoga*. Tirumūlar wrote extensively on *aṣṭāṅga yoga* as did Babaji's *guru*, Boganathar (Pōkanāthar). In reviving the ancient scientific art of *kriyā yoga* in the nineteenth century, Babaji undoubtedly drew much from Patañjali's *sūtras*. The many parallels between Babaji's *kriyā yoga* and the *sūtras*, as indicated in these commentaries, indicate that Patañjali was one of Babaji's sources.

1. *tapas svādhyāya-īśvara-praṇidhānā kriyā-yogaḥ*

tapas = intense practice; glowing, straightening by fire; "the burning away of the burden of one's *karma*"

svādhyāya = self-study

īśvara = the Lord, the Supreme Being

praṇidhāna = surrender to, devotion to (see I.23, II.45)

kriyā = action with awareness

yoga = union (see I.1)

Intense practice, self-study and devotion to the Lord constitute *kriyā yoga.*

Tapas means "intense practice." It comes from the verbal root *tap,* to make hot. It refers to any intense or prolonged practice for Self-realization, which involves overcoming the natural tendencies of the body, emotions or mind. Because of the resistance of the body, emotions or mind, heat or pain may develop as a bi-product, but this is never the objective. We may be learned in the sacred texts, or we may have performed many devotional acts, but if we have not performed *tapas,* the senses, mind and emotions will ultimately overwhelm our consciousness:

> In fear they ran from the croc' in the river
> And on the bank they fell into the embrace of the bear
> Thus are they the ignorant of scriptures
> Who from austere *tapas* run away
> For food and in hunger roam forever. (TM 1642)

Control of the senses is not an end in itself:

> In oneness of mind I did *tapas*
> And witnessed Lord's triumphant Feet;
> In eagerness of quest I did *tapas*
> And witnessed *Śiva* State;
> That alone is *tapas*
> That you perform in the yearning of the heart;
> What avails the *tapas* of those
> Who thus perform not? (TM 1636)

Self-study (*svādhyāya),* is not the mere study of sacred texts, but includes the observation of one's own behavior as well as the psychodynamics of the mind. This may take the form of recording of experiences in a journal, which permits us to transform what was a subjective experience into an objective one. As a result we become aware of what remains: the Seer (*draṣṭa,* see verse I.3). Gradually one ceases to identify with the personality, the sum of mental movements and habitual reactions. Self-study (*svādhyāya)* brings discrimination and self-mastery. *Siddhas* like Patañjali aspired not simply for transcendence, but also transformation of the lower human nature. There is no sharper sword than a spiritual diary to detect "the big thief", or the mind, which has snatched the "pearl of the Self." The mind gives us so many worries and delusions. One must not be lenient with it; check it unceasingly. Recording observations about oneself in a spiritual diary helps to do this, and provides us an opportunity to correct the daily mistakes. It also gives solace and inspiration.

The study of sacred texts also feeds and reminds us of what we truly are, and so helps us to grow.

Iśvara praṇidhāna or "surrender to the Lord" includes the cultivation of unconditional love for the Lord, as well as letting go of what disturbs us. Equanimity ultimately follows. One "let's go, and let's God." (See commentary on verses I.23 and II.45)

Kriyā Yoga is derived from the verbal root *kṛ* meaning "to do" or "to make," and is related to *karma*, the principle that every action brings about a reaction. Patañjali's *yoga* is therefore a three-fold path: intense practice (*tapas)*, self-study (*svādhyāya*) and devotion to the Lord (*īśvara-praṇidhāna*). In the first chapter, verses I.12 to I.16, Patañjali elaborates on the first of these three. He tells us that consistent repeated practice (*abhyāsa*) and detachment (*vairāgya*) are the means of *Yoga*.

It is interesting to note that Patañjali does not specify what we should practice constantly, that is, what specific techniques, except for detachment (*vairāgya)*. There is strong evidence to suggest that if one were to practice detachment continuously for at least three months, letting go of all disturbing mental and emotional reactions, one would reach the state of enlightenment, the supreme awakening of the mind. Ramana Maharshi described this supreme state of *samādhi* in the following words: "now nothing can disturb me anymore." As few persons are naturally endowed with much inclination towards consistent repeated practice (*abhyāsa*) and detachment (*vairāgya*), Patañjali prescribes preliminary practices in the second chapter. Feuerstein has pointed out, however, that Patañjali's *Yoga* was not the *aṣṭāṅga* or "eight-limbed" *Yoga*, described in verse II.28 to III.8, as has been commonly thought by most translators. Textual analysis has revealed that these verses were merely quoted from another unknown source.**(1)** There are frequent references to *aṣṭāṅga yoga* in the *Śaivāgamas*, and some of these works are older than Patañjali's *Sūtras*. Feuerstein has created the following tree diagram, which shows the relationship between the two branches of Patañjali's *Kriyā Yoga*:(2)

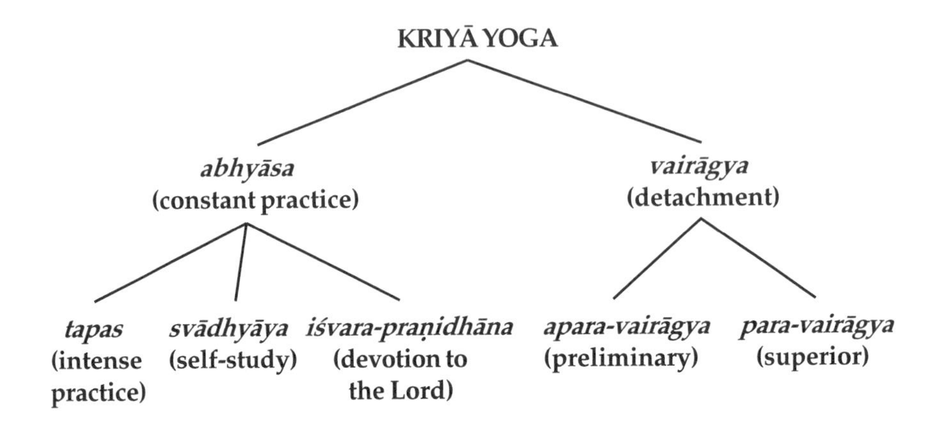

Practice: Practice intense practice *(tapas)*: set aside extended periods of time for concentrated and continuous practice of all forms of *Yoga*. Gradually increase the time up to 24 hours during days reserved exclusively for *Yoga*. On other days, practice ś*huddhi* or the *nityānanda kriyās* with increasing frequency. Develop equanimity in the face of the pain and pleasure, gain and loss, and other dualities.

Practice: Practice self-study *(svādhyāya)*: record your meditations in a journal; keep a spiritual diary, where you include observations about habits. Study sacred texts, including the Patañjali's *Sūtras* and *Tirumantiram*.

Practice: Practice devotion to the Lord (iś*vara-praṇidhāna*): cultivate surrender to, and love for, the Lord, as described in the commentary on verse I.23. External ceremonies are not as important as internal worship, as in the fourth breath control *kriyā (*a *prāṇāyāma kriyā* as taught in Babaji's *Kriya Yoga* level I initiation*)*, and in cultivating reverence for the Divine Presence in all.

2. *samādhi-bhāvana-arthaḥ kleśa-tanū-karaṇa-arthaś-ca*

samādhi = cognitive absorption

bhāvana = cultivating, causing to be, manifesting

arthaḥ = purpose, goal, end and aim

kleśa = affliction

tanū = lessened, diminished, weakened

karaṇa = doing, making, causing

arthaḥ = purpose, goal

ca = and

[They are used] for the purpose of weakening [any] affliction [and] cultivating cognitive absorption.

Before we can reach the goal of *Yoga*, cognitive absorption (*samādhi*), one must cleanse the fluctuations of consciousness *(cittavṛttiḥ)*, which were earlier defined as afflicted (*kliṣṭāḥ)* or non-afflicted (*akliṣṭāḥ)* (see verse I.5). It is a long process usually, but even a little practice will remove the cause of much suffering, as discussed in the following verses. *Kriyā Yoga* cleanses them of egoism, the habit of identifying with the body-mind complex. As they gradually become weaker, Self-realization dawns.

Practice: Do *sādhana* without pride, in a spirit of detachment (*vairāgya)*, to purify and eradicate the causes of suffering.

3. *avidyā-asmitā-rāga-dveṣa-abhiniveśāḥ pañca-kleśāḥ*

avidyā = ignorance

asmitā = egoism; "I-am-ness"

rāga = attachment

dveṣa = aversion; hatred; repulsion

abhiniveśāḥ = clinging to life; desire for continuity

pañcakleśāḥ = five afflictions

Ignorance, egoism, attachment, aversion and clinging to life are the five afflictions.

Here Patañjali enumerates the five afflictions, which prevent Self-realization. In the following verses he will explain each of them. The order in which they are presented is significant. Because of ignorance of our true Self, the ego arises; the ego, being the habit of identifying with the thoughts and sensations, creates attachments and aversion (likings and dislikings) and ultimately the fear of death.

Compare these with the five primal fetters *(pañca-pāśāḥ)*, which bind the individual soul, referred to repeatedly in *Tirumantiram*:

1. *tirodayi* (*tam.*) the power of confusion (literally 'concealment');
2. *āṇava (tam.)*: egoism;
3. *mayeyam (tam.)*: desires, the tangible manifestation of maya;
4. *māyā*: the material cause of the union of the conscious with the unconscious;
5. *karma*: a power, which by its continuity and development determines the nature and eventuality of the soul's repeated existences.

Practice: Meditate on the nature of these afflictions (*kleśāḥ*). Identify them by category. Prepare a detailed description of how each of them manifests in your life.

4. *avidyā kṣetram-uttareṣāṃ prasupta-tanu-vicchinna-udārāṇām*

avidyā = ignorance

kṣetraṁ = field, origin

uttareṣāṁ = of the others

prasupta = dormant, fallen, asleep

tanu = weak, attenuated, lessened, asleep

vicchinna = intercepted, suppressed, overpowered

udārāṇāṁ = active, engaged, aroused

Ignorance is the field [from which other] afflictions [arise] and can be dormant, weak, intercepted or active.

The primary cause of suffering is ignorance (*avidyā),* and it brings about the others. It refers not to ignorance in general, but specifically to an absence of Self-awareness. It is the cause of the confusion between the subject, "I am," and all objects of awareness. It hides our inner awareness and creates a false identity: I am the body, mind, senses, emotions, etc.

In the case of the average person, ignorance (*avidyā),* egoism (*asmitā*), attachment (*rāga*), aversion (*dveṣa)* and clinging to life (*abhiniveśaḥ)* are constant and sustained. We constantly follow the prompting of the subconscious based desires. When our well-being, or survival, is threatened we typically respond in fear without any reflection. When we begin to practice *Yoga,* however, we intercept many such promptings, resist them and substitute feelings of love, self-discipline, generosity (*dāna),* etc. It requires vigilance and effort however; if not, the old habits are revived.

In an advanced practitioner of Yoga, the afflictions (*kleśāḥ)* become very weak (*prasuptāḥ),* or dormant, because he or she no longer responds to them. The practitioner's constant discipline (*sādhana*) has resulted in a state of equanimity, which cannot be disturbed by such promptings.

Practice: After identifying the affliction, begin to give up one habit, or desire, at a time. Notice how your experience in eliminating them evolves through stages. In the first stage, one makes no effort to eliminate them; in the second stage, one begins to exert effort; in the third stage, one brushes temptations aside nearly effortlessly. In the fourth stage they remain only at the level of the subconscious, suppressed. In these later stages one may encounter them only during dreams while sleeping.

5. *anitya-aśuci-duḥkha-anātmasu nitya-śuci-sukha-ātma-khyātir-avidyā*

anitya = impermanent

aśuci = impure

duḥkha = painful

anātmasu = in non-Self, concerning or regarding non-self

nitya = permanent, eternal, continual

śuci = pure, untainted

sukha = pleasant, happiness, well-being

ātman = Self

khyātiḥ = cognition

avidyā = ignorance

Ignorance is seeing the impermanent as permanent, the impure as pure, the painful as pleasurable and the non-Self as the Self.

This is the fundamental error to which humans are prone, and involves the mistaken sense of identity with what we are not. We say: "I am tired" or "I am sick, angry or worried." We approach the truth, however, when we say: "my body is tired," or "I have angry thoughts." Our current cultural context, the media, our language syntax and our educational system all foster this fundamental error, which hides our true identity, the Self. The Self is the eternal witness, the Seer, a constant, pure One Being, infinite, all pervasive, present in everything. Everything else is changing and will therefore be lost one day. By clinging to the impermanent, to what changes, we ignore the Real, and we suffer. All desire is painful for it creates an insatiable need to have something, which we currently do not possess, or to be something, which we are not. Even when we fulfill desires there will always be more desires, as well as the desire not to lose what we have, hence more suffering.

Practice: Perceive the permanent, pure Self, which pervades everything. Abide in That.

6. *dṛg-darśana-śaktyor-eka-ātmatā-iva-asmitā*

dṛg = (dṛś) Seer

darśana = what is seen; correct understanding; here: instrument of seeing

śaktyor = of the two powers (*śakti*)

ekātmata = identity; singular nature or self; "having the quality of self-ness"

iva = as it were; as though

asmitā = egoism; "I-am-ness"

Egoism is the identification, as it were, of the powers of the Seer [Purusha] with that of the instrument of seeing [body-mind].

Egoism (*asmitā*) is the habit of identifying with what we are not: the body-mind-personality, the instrument of cognition. We falsely identify with thoughts, sensations and emotions without recognizing that they are objects only, merely reflections of our awareness. This leads to the individuation of our consciousness: "I-am-ness" and its confusion with "I am the body," "I am this feeling," etc. This subject-object confusion is removed by the practice of detachment and discernment. This error is a product of our basic ignorance as to who we truly are.

Practice: Feel that you are not "the doer," but only the Seer. Be a witness and an instrument and notice how everything gets done. When things go well, thank the Lord. When things go badly, take responsibility and learn to do better.

7. *sukha-anuśayī rāgaḥ*

sukham = pleasure

anuśayīn = clinging to, resting on

rāgaḥ = attachment

Attachment is the clinging to pleasure.

Because of the individuation of consciousness, and its false identification with a particular body and set of thoughts and memories, we are attracted to various pleasant experiences in our environment. Attachment *(rāgaḥ)*, like fear, springs from the imagination (*vikalpa)*. It occurs when we confuse the internal experience of bliss *(ānanda)* with a set of outer circumstances, or factors, and we call this association pleasure (*sukham)*. We imagine that pleasure depends upon the presence of these external circumstances, or factors. When they are no longer there, we experience attachment, the delusion that the inner joy cannot return unless we again possess the external factors. Attachment involves clinging (*anuśayī)*, and of course, suffering (*duḥkhaṁ)*. Even when we possess the external factors, we may still experience attachment because of the fear (imagination) of losing it. However, in reality, bliss is self-existent, unconditional and independent of external circumstances or factors. One need only be aware to experience it.

Practice: (1) Cultivate awareness before, during, and after pleasurable activities or circumstances. Notice that bliss remains throughout, as long as awareness is present. (2) Practice letting go of feelings of attachment.

8. *duḥkha-anuśayī dveṣaḥ*

duḥkha = suffering

anuśayīn = clinging to; resting on

dveṣa = aversion

Aversion is clinging to suffering.

In the same way, we are repulsed by various experiences in our environment. These are relative terms, and what is painful for one, may be pleasant for another person. There is a third possible response however, detachment (*vairāgya)*, which Patañjali proposes as the key practice for going beyond the painful and pleasurable (see verse I.12, 15).

When we go deep within, standing back from a painful experience, its cause becomes evident. By cultivating this perspective and understanding, as well as patience and tolerance, we are no longer troubled. "If it costs our peace of mind, it costs too much." Changing an outer painful situation is often impossible, without first changing our perception of it. We should first focus our will on clearing and deepening our consciousness to avoid reacting with aversion. Aspire for an outer change, for a more harmonious situation. Accept any work that has been given to you in the spirit of *karma yoga* (selfless service), as spiritual training, to purify you of attachment (*rāga)* and aversion (*dveṣa).*

Practice: Perform all actions selflessly, skillfully and patiently, recognizing that you are not the "doer." Cultivate equanimity as you perform actions, and with regard to the results.

9. *sva-rasa-vāhī viduṣo' pi tathā-rūḍho' bhiniveśaḥ*

svarasa = own inclination; literally 'own juice or essence'

vāhī = carried; supported

viduṣo pi = even the wise

tathā = thus

rūḍhaḥ = arisen, produced

abhiniveśaḥ = clinging to life; desire for continuity

Clinging to life [which] is self-sustaining, arises even in the wise.

This is the basic drive of self-preservation, the fundamental will to live, which exists in all living beings. It is an instinct, and is based upon the fear of death and false identification with the body. We have had to go through the painful process of death and rebirth so many times, that we shrink from having to repeat it. Once we realize we are the immortal Self, we can free ourselves from all of these afflictions (*kleśāḥ)*.

Practice: Reflect on this statement: "to die unto death, to become incapable of dying because death has no more reality."

10. *te pratiprasava-heyāḥ sūkṣmāḥ*

te = these (refers to afflictions)

pratiprasava = resolving back into their cause; tracing causes back to their origin

heyāḥ = destroyed; overcome

sūkṣmāḥ = subtle

These [afflictions in their] subtle [form], are destroyed by tracing [their] cause[s] back to [their] origin.

The five afflictions (*pañca-kleśāḥ*) maintain our false identity and separation from the Self. Patañjali tells us that they can be removed on two levels in verse II.10 and II.11. On the subtle level, they exist as subconscious impressions (*saṁskāras*), and can be eliminated only by the repeated return to our source through the various stages of samadhi. Because the subconscious impressions are not accessible to us in ordinary consciousness, or even meditation, one must eliminate their root, egoism, by repeatedly identifying with our true Self. The little "i" becomes subsumed gradually in the greater "I" and as it does, the subconscious impressions dissolve.

It is significant that Patañjali does not advocate cruder methods, such as "ego-crushing" behavior by a spiritual teacher, nor even argumentation, reasoning or emotion-based approaches. He only advocates resolving the afflictions (*kleśāḥ)* back into their primal cause, which as shown in verse II.4, is the "ignorance" (the absence of Self-awareness, the confusion between the Seer and the Seen, the objects of awareness). In verse I.12, he has prescribed the means to do this: constant practice and detachment. Ask yourself, "Who is attached?"

"Who feels aversion?" "Who is it that says "I", "My", "Mine?" Such thoughts and feelings do not belong to you. Let them go.

It is the ego that feels guilt and pride. It is the ego that feels guilt over some actions, which it sees as bad, and therefore feels unworthy. It is the ego, which thinks it is doing the practices and thinks it is itself releasing us of our ego. It is the ego, which thinks "I" cannot do the practices, cannot meditate, or control my emotions or habits. A strong ego makes us wallow in the misery of guilt. The ego is the sense of being the doer and of being in charge of our lives. In fact, the ego feels that if it weren't in charge, we could not survive. By doing *sādhana,* focusing on the Self, one begins to see that Nature does everything, and that ego never did anything. But first, we must deal with the grosser level of mental fluctuations, arising within consciousness, as he describes in the next verse.

11. *dhyāna-heyās-tad-vṛttayaḥ*

dhyāna = meditation

heyāḥ = destroyed

tad = these, those

vṛittayaḥ = fluctuations [arising within consciousness]

[In the active state], these fluctuations [arising within consciousness] are destroyed by meditation.

This indicates that the elimination of the fluctuations arising within consciousness (see verses I.2 and I.5) is a pre-requisite for cognitive absorption (*samādhi).* They can be eliminated by the practice of meditation (*dhyāna),* which may be defined in Verse III.2 as "the experience of having the mind fixed on one object only (*pratyaya-ekatānatā dhyānam).*"

Meditation *(dhyāna)* is the easiest process of the human mind, but narrow in results. Continuous awareness is more difficult, but greater in results. Self-observation and liberation from the chains of thought is the most difficult of all, but greatest in its results. One can choose one or all of these methods, each in its own place and for its own object. This requires firm faith, patience, and a great energy of Will in the self-application of *Yoga*.

Practice: Meditate to understand the Self. Practice continuous awareness to experience the Self. And observe yourself to see what must go, in order for you to become the Self.

12. *kleśa-mūlaḥ karma-āśayo dṛṣṭa-adṛṣṭa-janma-vedanīyaḥ*

kleśaḥ = affliction

mūlaḥ = the root, foundation

karma-āśayaḥ = the reservoir of karmas

dṛṣṭa = seen or present

adṛṣṭa = unseen or future

janma = birth, existence, life, birth

vedanīyaḥ = to be felt or experienced

The reservoir of *karmas* rooted in the afflictions, is experienced in seen [present] and unseen [future] existence.

Because of the existence of the *kleśāḥ*, the afflictions of ignorance (*avidyā*), egoism *(asmitā)*, attachment (*rāga)* aversion (*dveṣa*) and the clinging to life *(abhiniveśaḥ)* we accumulate and express *karmas*. There are three types of *karma*:

1. *prārabdha karma*: those presently being expressed and exhausted through this birth;
2. *āgama karma*: new karmas being created during this birth;
3. *saṁjita karma*: those waiting to be fulfilled in future births;

The receptacle for all the karmas is known as the *karma-āśaya*, "the reservoir, or womb, of karma" or "action-deposit."

The *karmas* wait for an opportunity to come to the surface and to express themselves through the *kleśāḥ*. One strong *karma* may call for a particular birth and body to express itself, and other closely related karmas will also be expressed or exhausted through it. This goes on until one attains Self-realization and ceases to create new *karmas*.

We need to understand that we are simply living out our karmic destiny. Time is *karma*, the sages say. We have our own karmic map. We also need to understand that each person has his own *karma* and acts according to it. We wonder why someone acts a certain way, or lives a certain way. He is wondering the same about us. Each of us is programmed with a certain nature. Our opinions of what is perfection come from what we were taught and how well we have learned our lessons. The circumstances of our life occur because of our *karma*. But we have free will as to how we will deal with these, positively or negatively. If we choose to deal with these negatively, for example, in creating suffering for others, the reactions return to us in more intense or terrible forms. Dealing with circumstances patiently, creating happiness for others, neutralizes the karmic consequences gradually.

Practice: Reflect on this statement: "To break free of *karma* we must realize that we have already attained what we are seeking."

13. *sati mūla tad-vipāko jāty-āyus-bhogā*

sati = being, existing, ocurring

mūla = root

tad = that, this

vipākaḥ = fruits

jāti = birth, production,

āyuḥ = life span, vital power, life

bhogāḥ = experiences, enjoyments, eating

So long as the root exists, [its] fruits also exist; [namely] birth, and [its] experiences.

So long as the mind maintains attractions and aversions, the individual soul will continue to take birth in order to fulfill its karmic deposits. If one wants to eat excessively, the *karma* may better express itself in a pig's body. The person's soul will continue to evolve through the experience of a pig's body. It is not the body, or senses, which seek to experience various pleasures or to avoid pain, but the mind, driven by its *kleśāḥ* and karmic deposits. The span of life *(āyuḥ)* and types of experience *(bhogaḥ)* in a particular birth *(jāti)* are determined by one's reservoir of karma *(karma-āśayaḥ).* When some *karmas* are exhausted, the soul seeks to express remaining ones. We can see this occurring whenever our life takes a new turn, for example, a midlife crisis, or major career change.

Liberation is being free from *karma* and *saṁskāras.* It does not mean the end of physical life, although it may end your playing certain parts in the play. It may mean you play a new part. But you will be totally aware that you are simply playing a part, which will allow you freedom to play it with unconditional love and truth.

Practice: Repeat: "Lord, I accept the situation as it is." Then be still, and without thinking about it, do what must be done, with unconditional love and dedication to truth. Do your duty in the spirit of selfless service (*karma yoga)* skillfully, and without attachment to the fruits. Cultivate equanimity and awareness.

14. *te hlāda-paritāpa-phalāḥ puṇya-apuṇya-hetutvāt*

te = they, these

hlāda = pleasure, joy, delight

paritāpa = pain, grief, sorrow

phalāḥ = fruits, consequence, result

puṇya = meritorious, favourable, virtuous

apuṇya = non-meritorious, unfavourable, non-virtuous

hetutvāt = because of the cause; because of the motive

Because of virtuous and non-virtuous *karma*, there are [corresponding] pleasurable and painful consequences.

If we bring happiness (*hlāda)* to others we gain pleasure; if we bring suffering (*haritāpa)* to others we will reap pain for ourselves. If we allow true happiness for ourselves, we automatically make others who are near us happier - whether or not they know that initially. Our habits, or subconscious impressions (*saṁskāras)*, largely determine our actions. Therefore the quality of our birth (*jāti)*, lifespan *(ayuḥ)* and life experience (*bhogaḥ)* is determined by our subconscious impressions *(saṁskāras)*. Therefore we should cultivate thoughts, words and deeds, which will be edifying to ourselves, and to others.

Practice: Cultivate thoughts, words and deeds, which will be edifying for yourself and others, but first listen to and reflect on your innermost guidance, and avoid egoistic reactions.

15. *pariṇāma-tāpa-saṃskāra-duḥkhair-guṇa-vṛtti-virodhāc-ca duḥkham-eva sarvaṃ vivekinaḥ*

pariṇāma = transformation, change

tāpa = anxiety; sorrow

saṃskāra = subconscious impressions; impression left by previous action

duḥkhair = by or with pains, sufferings

guṇa = quality

vṛittiḥ = fluctuations [of consciousnss]

virodhāt = because of a conflict or opposition

ca = and

duḥkha = pain; suffering

eva = indeed, thus

sarva = all

vivekinaḥ = of discrimination or discerning

Because of the conflict between the fluctuations [of consciousness] and the constituent forces of nature, and with the suffering [that arises from] the subconscious impressions, anxiety and change, for the discriminating person, indeed all is sorrowful.

Even getting what we want creates suffering *(duḥkha)* when we begin to fear losing it, or when the habit of craving it leads to more craving *(tṛṣṇa)*, fear *(bhaya)* and anxiety *(tāpa)*. While we may have moments of pleasure, they are bound to end, and the knowledge of this creates anxiety, fear and suffering. No experience gives everlasting happiness. When we realize this, we begin to discern the source of lasting happiness as lying beyond attachment to things or persons. It is not the experience of pleasurable things which creates suffering, but the attachment to them. So the wise allow things to come, or to go, without becoming lost in thoughts of fear, or anxiety, or attachment. The wise cultivate detachment *(vairāgya)* in order to end the habit of attachment and the confusion between well-being and external objects or circumstances.

Practice: Let go of feelings of sorrow, neediness, fear and anxiety as they arise in daily life. Feel the relief that comes when you fully release such feelings.

16. *heyaṃ duḥkham-anāgatam*

heya = eliminated, overcome, destroyed

duḥkha = sorrow; pain

anāgatam = future

[That which is] to be eliminated is future sorrow.

We do not have to suffer to be happy! While it is obvious when put this way, the presence of our conditioning, in the form of the subconscious impressions *(saṁskāras)* and the five causes of affliction *(pañca-kleśāḥ)*, keeps us in a state of amnesia regarding this truism. So *Yoga* is the ultimate reminder or "antidote" for our human forgetfulness. Only when we remember the Self can we go beyond the "sorrow yet to come" (*duḥkham-anāgatam)*, which results from our reservoir of *karma (karma-āśaya).* Seeking only pleasure, we forget that everything in time and space will eventually pass; so pleasure seeking inevitably leads to sorrow. Cultivating inner awareness, we find bliss (*ānanda)*, even when life delivers karmically a truckload of rotten tomatoes! We stand back from the drama, and note: "Ah, look at that!"

Practice: Make a list of things that in your heart you know need to be avoided. Ask yourself if any of these things are in your nature to do. If you have done any of the things on the list, what was the result? Be non-judgmental.

17. *draṣṭṛ-dṛśyayoḥ saṃyogo heya-hetuḥ*

draṣṭṛ = the Seer

dṛśyayoḥ = the seen, those [two which] are visible

saṃyoga = union

heya = eliminated, destroyed; overcome

hetu = cause, reason, motive

The cause [of suffering] to be eliminated is the union of the Seer and the Seen.

When our body feels some pain or we have experienced a loss, we say, "I am suffering." We confuse the Self *(puruṣa)* who sees *(dṛśya)*, with the constituent forces of nature (*prakṛti*), everything else. Ask yourself: "who suffers?" You will immediately realize that it is not you. You are only the observer. Misplaced identity is the root cause of suffering. The union of the Seer and the Seen (*draṣṭṛ-dṛśyayoḥ saṃyogaḥ)* is apparent only.

Or, from another perspective, really feel the pain, until you come out on the other side. Be with it completely. It is your greatest teacher, however you will never know that if you do not feel it entirely.

We came here to knowingly or unknowingly participate in the union between the Seer and the Seen. If the body must undergo certain experiences according to its *karma,* then the only way to avoid the inevitable sorrow is to balance Spirit and Will. Nature sees that you have equal parts of pleasure and sorrow. When we can merge our personal will with Divine Will we can accept both joy and sorrow equally. The experiences that come to us are the experiences we need at the time.

Practice: Accept sorrow and joy equally. Sit still and give both sorrow and joy to the Supreme Being.

18. *prakāśa-kriyā-sthiti-śīlaṃ bhūta-indriya-ātmakaṃ bhoga-apavarga-arthaṃ dṛśyam*

prakāśa = brightness, light, lustre

kriyā = activity

sthiti = inertia, remaining inert

śīlaṃ = nature, quality, character

bhūta = element, constituent of the manifest world

indriya = sense organ

ātmakaṁ = having the self-nature of; consists of

bhoga = experience

apavarga = liberation

artham = purpose

dṛśyaṁ = the Seen

The Seen is of the quality of brightness, activity and inertia; and

consists of the elements and sense organs whose purpose is [to provide both] experience and liberation [to the Self].

This aphorism defines the constituent forces of Nature (*prakṛti),* the Seen *(dṛśya).* It includes everything capable of becoming the object of the transcendental subject or Self. Nature's three principal modes of manifestation correspond to the three primary constituents of Nature (*tri-guṇas*). Brightness or equilibrium accompanies the constituent known as *sattva..* Activity or movement accompanies the *guṇa* of *rajas* and inertia or denseness accompanies *tamas.* These three modes occur at both the material and psychological levels. Nature provides us with experience and ultimately liberates our consciousness from its bondage of false identification. Eventually we feel we have had enough suffering in the hands of Nature and seek a way out of egoistic confusion ("I am the body-mind," etc). Nature includes the elements and our own bodies, mind and emotions. It is continually changing. With detachment and discernment we learn to go beyond it. Liberation of the Self from the bonds of ignorance (see verse II.3) occurs as we learn from the experiences given to us in Nature.

Practice: Practice the *dhyāna kriyās,* taught in Babaji's *Kriya Yoga,* which involve the five senses. Fully understand and appreciate the senses and sensual experience. Treat all experiences as an opportunity to practice awareness, to be the Seer, and to detach from identification with the Seen, the objects of experience.

19. *viśeṣa-aviśeṣa-liṅga-mātra-aliṅgāni guṇa-parvāṇi*

viśheṣha = specific; distinct

aviśeṣha = non-specific; indistinct

liṅgamātra = defined

aliṅga = undefinable

guṇa = the primary constituents of nature

parvāṇi = divisions

The divisions of the primary constituent forces of nature are specific, non-specific, defined and undefinable.

Patañjali analyzes Nature. At the subtlest level it is in a static, indefinable state; then when it begins to manifest it can be defined. Then it forms into the subtle sense objects, perceived by the mind and intellect (as visual images or ideas, for example). Finally, it manifests at the material level as gross objects, which we can sense through the five sense organs. Normally our understanding requires that we first apprehend with one of our physical senses, but in *Yoga*, as the intuition and subtle senses develop, we may apprehend such extrasensory phenomena as auras or activities occurring at a distance, or events occurring in the future.

Unlike other *siddhas* and *tantrikas*, Patañjali does not describe Nature as power (*śakti)*, the Divine Mother or any other feminine, or personal, form or power.

The *siddhas* were first-rate scientists, and they recorded and applied their observations about Nature in many fields of knowledge, including medicine, botany, alchemy and physics.

Practice: Contemplate how nature manifests at all levels, as indicated by the findings of the physical and social sciences. Seek inspiration by doing research in these fields. Contribute to human understanding of the Nature of things. Practice the *dhyāna kriyās* involving the five senses as taught in Babaji's *Kriya Yoga* initiations.

20. *draṣṭā dṛśi-mātraḥ śuddho' pi pratyaya-anupaśyaḥ*

draṣṭā = the Seer (see I.3)

dṛśi = the power of seeing

mātraḥ = only, merely

śuddhaḥ = pure, correct, cleansed

api = also, even, used as an emphatic
pratyaya = awareness; here: thoughts

anupaśyaḥ = perceiving

[Being] pure, the Seer, through the power of merely seeing [directly] perceives thoughts.

The Seer is the Self (see verse I.3) the pure subject that transcends. It witnesses continuously the movements arising within itself, the mind. While the mind has many different discontinuous experiences through the five senses, emotions, memory, etc., the Self remains constant. The mind is its object. The Seer appears to see through the mind, but in reality the seeing of the Seer is independent of what the mind experiences.

Our thoughts and ideas sometimes become an obstacle or a complication to the Divine Will. The best thing for us to do is to open to that Will. By being consciously still and peaceful, we allow Divine Wisdom to flow freely through us.

Practice: Sit still, letting go of all thoughts of doing, being, or having and turn over absolutely everything to the Lord.

21. *tad-artha eva dṛśyasya-ātmā*

tadartha = for [the *puruṣa*'s) sake

eva = only

dṛśya = the seen *prakṛti*

ātman = the Self

The Seen [exists] only for the sake of the Self.

With reference to verse II.18, the Seen exists only to serve the Self's liberation. Once the Seer is liberated from its confusion with the Seen, the Seen serves no further purpose. The Seer is just a witness, not a doer nor an enjoyer. Until then, the Seen gives experience and by such experience we gradually wake up from the dream that we are the Seen. Those *siddhas* who remain on the physical plane indefinitely do so to assist the liberation of others.

Practice: Clearly distinguish the Seer from the Seen, and abide only as the Seer. Appreciate how the Seen provides us with so many opportunities to learn this distinction and to completely liberate the Seer.

22. *kṛta-arthaṃ prati naṣṭam-apy-anaṣṭaṃ tad-anya-sādhāraṇatvāt*

kṛta = done

arthaṁ = purpose, goal

prati = towards, for

naṣṭa = destroyed, disappeared, lost

api = even though

anaṣṭam = not destroyed

tad = that

anya = other

sādhāraṇatvāt = because of, due to commonality, universality

For one who has attained the goal [of liberation, the Seen] disappears [yet, the seen] is not destroyed because of its common universality.

This aphorism rejects the notion that the world exists only in our minds, but in reality does not exist. Patañjali herein asserts that external objects do have their independent existence and they are not affected by our Self-realization. Self-realization is an individual event, which does not annihilate the objective world. This is in contrast to the teachings of many schools of *Vedānta,* which holds that Nature (*prakṛti*) is illusion (*māyā),* with no objective reality. *Śaiva Siddhānta, Kashmiri Śaivism* and *Tantric Śaktism* all agree that the "world or the seen, is a reality."

We can only serve others by being our Selves. We can only love others for the sake of the Self. Clearly distinguish the Self in others from their behavior. We may not love their behavior, and still love their Selves. They are usually "dreaming with their eyes open" as the *siddhas* described our human condition.

Practice: See the Seer in everyone. Relate to them as they truly are, not who they think they are. Treat everyone and everything with reverence.

23. *sva-svāmi-śaktyoḥ sva-rūpa-upalabdhi-hetuḥ saṃyogaḥ*

sva = own; here: owned (*prakṛti*)

svāmi = the Owner (*puruṣa*); lord, chief

śaktyoḥ = [two] power(s), energy, ability

svarūpa = essence; own form; nature (see I.3)

upalabdhi = recognition; perception

hetu = cause

saṁyoga = union

The union of owner [*puruṣa*] and owned [*prakṛti*] causes the recognition of the essence and power of them both.

Through the world of Nature *(prakṛti),* which includes our senses, mind and feelings, we come to know our Self. So Nature is not just what hides our Self; it is ultimately our Mother teacher guiding us home. The state of union between *(saṁyoga)* the two enables a contrast, which is ultimately instructive for us.

Practice: Be calmly active and actively calm, established in Being, as a witness to all of Nature's activities. Realize that you are not the doer. Learn and practice the *kriyā* of continual bliss (*nityānanda kriyā)* as learned in *Babaji's Kriya Yoga* level II initiation.

24. *tasya hetur-avidyā*

tasya = its; of it

hetu = cause; reason, motive

avidyā = ignorance

The cause of this union is ignorance.

The false identification of our Self with the objects of experience is not illusionary, but it is based upon ignorance (*avidyā).* Once we realize our error we can say "How ignorant I was!" Self-realization is the solution to our ignorance.

<u>Practice</u>: Remind your mind that it is not the "subject". Stand back from it and remain firm as the inner Seer.

25. *tad-abhāvāt saṃyoga-abhāvo hānaṃ tad-dṛśeḥ kaivalyam*

tad = that (refers to ignorance)

abhāvāt = because of, due to absence or non-existence

saṃyoga = union

abhāvaḥ = non-existence, absence, negation

hānaṁ = removal, absence, decline

tad = that

dṛśeḥ = from the Seen

kaivalyaṁ = absolute freedom (see IV.34), absolute unity, beatitude, detachment from all other connections; aloneness.

Without this ignorance [*avidyā*], no such union [*saṁyoga*] occurs. This is the absolute freedom [*kaivalyam*] from the Seen [*dṛśeḥ*].

Who suffers? Who is happy? Who am I? When we answer these

questions we see that we are only the witness, pure awareness. Thus we are absolutely free, but alone. The Seer abides in his own true form (*svarūpa,* see verse I.3). The Seer's *karma* unfolds but the Seer is unaffected by it, remaining as a detached witness to the drama of life.

Practice: Make all events, thoughts and emotions the object of awareness and so remain as the Seer. Learn and practice *nityānanda kriyā.*

26. *viveka-khyātir-aviplavā hāna-upāyaḥ*

viveka = discrimination, discerning

khyāti = perception, knowledge

aviplava = uninterrupted, unbroken, unwavering

hāna = removal, absence, decline; escape

upāya = method, means by which one attains a goal

Uninterrupted discriminative discernment is the method for its removal.

How are we to remove this ignorance (*avidyā*) and reach Self-realization? Patañjali advises us to distinguish what is permanent from what is transitory; the Real from the relatively unreal, the Self as distinct from the world. We take the perspective of a witness and train the inner consciousness to gradually withdraw, to stand back even from our own mental processes. In the final stage of this discernment, we identify with the Self in non-distinguished cognitive absorption (*asaṁprajñātaḥ samādhi*). Feuerstein refers to this as "the unceasing vision of discernment."**(3)** In order to grasp the Truth, moment to moment observation is necessary. Each of us must decide for ourselves what needs to be let go of, and what may stay.

Practice: From moment to moment, for increasing periods, practice being the witness, distinguishing the permanent from the transitory, the pure subject from all objects.

27. *tasya saptadhā prānta-bhūmiḥ prajñā*

tasya = his

saptadhā = sevenfold

prānta = final, last

bhūmi = ground, stage

prajñā = wisdom

One's wisdom in the final stage is sevenfold.

While Patañjali does not explain what is the "Seven-fold wisdom" (*saptadhā prajñā*). The Sage Vyāsa has identified it as follows: we experience the end of (1) desire to know anything more; (2) desire to stay away from anything; (3) desire to gain anything new; (4) desire to do anything; (5) sorrow; (6) fear; and (7) delusion.

These occur as we begin to abide in "our own true form or nature" (*svarūpa*):

1. We realize that the source of all wisdom is within ourselves. Our seeking for expressions of the truth outside ourselves comes to an end.
2. The cessation of pain occurs as our attachments (rāgāḥ) and aversions (dveṣāḥ) fall away.
3. In cognitive absorption (samādhi) all sense of individual separation or lack is gone. There is a sense of oneness with all.
4. We feel that we are no longer the doer; there is no attachment or individual selfish desire.
5. The ego subsides and the subconscious impressions can no longer disturb the mind.
6. The subconscious impressions fall away "like rocks fallen from a mountain peak, never to return."
7. The Self alone remains, resting in its own true form, or nature, completely peaceful, pure and alone. The illusion of identification with the mind is gone and we remain in cognitive absorption (samādhi) permanently.

Practice: As you notice mental or emotional disturbances arising throughout the day, ask yourself, whenever possible, "Now, can I let go of my need to know this, to have this, to do this, to be this, or to avoid this?" Then ask yourself: "Will I let it go?" and "When?" Feel the body-mind release the tension associated with holding onto it.

28. *yoga-aṅga-anuṣṭhānād-aśuddhi-kṣaye jñāna-dīptir-ā-viveka-khyāteḥ*

yoga = union

aṅga = limb

anuṣṭhāna = because, from or due to following an action or doing a practice

aśuddhi = impure

kṣaye = in or at the destruction, dwindling or loss

jñānadīpti = light of wisdom, knowledge

ā = up to, as far as

viveka = discrimination, discernment

khyāti = perception, knowledge.

By the practice of the limbs of Yoga, the impurities dwindle away and there dawns the light of wisdom leading to discriminative discernment.

This verse indicates that *Yoga*, as a system, existed long before the Patañjali *Sūtras*. It was handed down primarily as an oral tradition, but there are references to various systems of *Yoga* in earlier works, including the *Maitrāyaṇīya-Upaniṣad*. This verse reminds us that the practice of *aṣṭāṅga Yoga*, as described in the following verse, brings us to what was described in verse II.26.

The various limbs (*aṅga*) of *Yoga* are not an end in themselves: not a way to escape life, or to impress others with our form or skill. They serve us only when they serve to purify, to bring us wisdom (*prajñā*) and the "unceasing vision of discernment" (*asaṁprajñātaḥ samādhi).* But by being regular in our practice, we become a master of the body, breath and mind, and thus facilitate the liberation of the Self from the confusion of egoism and negative habits.

Practice: Do all your practices with full awareness, being the Seer, and not the doer.

29. *yama-niyama-āsana-prāṇāyāma-pratyāhāra-dhāraṇā-dhyāna-samādhayo' ṣṭāv-aṅgāni*

yama = restraint, self-control

niyama = observance

āsana = posture, position

prāṇāyāma = breath control

pratyāhāra = withdrawal of senses, retreat

dhāraṇā = concentration

dhyāna = meditation

samādhyayaḥ = (from *samādhi)* contemplations, absorptions or superconscious states

aṣṭau = eight

aṅgāni = limbs or parts

The eight limbs of Yoga are:

1. yama	*[restraint]*
2. niyama	*[observance]*
3. āsana	*[posture]*
4. prāṇāyāma	*[breath control]*

5. pratyāhāra	*[sense withdrawal]*
6. dhāraṇā	*[concentration]*
7. dhyāna	*[meditation]*
8. samādhi	*[cognitive absorption]*

This verse begins a new section which, according to Georg Feuerstein, was either added to later editions of the *Sūtras* or was a quotation by Patañjali from an unknown source.**(4)**

In *Tirumantiram* verse 549 Tirumūlar indicates that *Naṇḍi*, or *Śiva*, revealed the eightfold science of Yoga (*yoga aṣṭāṅga*). The eight limbs are the same as those in the *Sūtras* but *Tirumantiram* verses 549 to 631 presents these eight limbs much more completely and frankly than the *Sūtras*. Tirumūlar cannot be said to have borrowed his ideas from Patañjali. Tirumantiram goes the full length of *Yoga* as known in his time whereas Patañjali stops short of it.

While most commentators have interpreted these eight limbs as stages, to be practiced successively, at least one commentator **(5)** has recognized that this is not the case, but that they could be arranged in a circle: by their combined power the *yogin* propels himself along the path of internalization.

Compare this with the *Tirumantiram* verse 552:

> *Yama*, niyama and *āsana* numberless,
> *Prāṇāyāma* wholesome and *pratyāhāra* alike,
> Dhāraṇā, *dhyāna* and *samādhi* to triumph,
> These eight are the steely limbs of *Yoga*.

Modern students of Haṭha *Yoga* have been lead by contemporary scholars to believe that *Haṭha Yoga* was developed only during the early part of the second millennium, as referred to in the *Gheranda Saṁhitā*, and the *Haṭha Yoga Pradīpika*. This verse and TM verses 558-563 indicate at least 180 important *āsanas*.

In the following verses, each of these limbs is described by Patañjali.

Practice: Practice all limbs of *Yoga* as a system, wherein each complements and furthers the others.

30. *ahiṃsā-satya-asteya-brahmacarya-aparigrahā yamāḥ*

ahiṃsā = non-violence, absence of desire to kill or injure

satya = truthfulness; authenticity, sincerity

asteya = non-stealing

brahmacarya = chastity, sexual restraint

aparigrahāḥ = greedlessness; renunciation

yamāḥ = restraint

The restraints are non-violence, truthfulness, non-stealing, chastity and greedlessness.

Non-violence (*ahiṁsā)* includes non-harming, whether it be by action, words or thoughts. *Hiṁsā* means injury, so *ahiṁsā* is not to cause injury. Our words and thoughts have great power. They can harm others. They can stimulate harmful actions. When we cease to do harm to others, we find that the mind ceases to harbor resentment, envy, anger and fear. Consequently, our consciousness becomes purified. By cultivating forgiveness we can turn away such feelings, which harm not only others, but ultimately ourselves.

Truthfulness *(satya)* implies not only the avoidance of lying, but also exaggeration, deceit, pretending, hypocrisy and truth in advertising. Otherwise we deceive ourselves, postpone the working out of actual *karma,* and create or reinforce new karmic consequences. By leaving aside all fiction, all imaginary or unreal things, in mind, speech and action, one quickly discovers what is truth. To speak only what is true is very revealing. So much of what is spoken is so unnecessary, so trivial and unreal. To cultivate silence, or to speak only what is edifying, after reflection, brings great clarity to our minds and relationships.

Non-stealing (*asteya)* includes avoiding the taking of something that does not belong to oneself. Stealing engulfs our consciousness with darkness, wherein we fail to see our essential unity. It closes our heart, strengthens egoistic tendencies, and drives us away from the path of Self-realization. It is a manifestation of fear and weakness in the face of desire. By indulging it, we give up our power of self-control and strengthen the hold that negative forces may have upon us.

Chastity (*brahmacarya)*, involves sexual abstinence in the physical, emotional or vital, as well as mental planes. Its cultivation facilitates letting go of what is usually a great source of distraction and suffering for most persons, and consequently the process of Self-realization. Even if one lives in a committed relationship with a partner, if one can cultivate moderation and awareness in one's sexual relations, most distraction and dispersion can be avoided. One loves the other as one's Self. When a vow is observed incorrectly, there is the danger of suppression, and consequently, dangerous psychological effects. One must be careful not to develop antipathy towards members of the opposite sex, or feelings of guilt, shame, or frustration with regards to sexual impulses. In today's hedonistic culture, the ideal of sexual abstinence and purity will strike most people as not only odd, but also impossible. It is neither. However, it may be necessary for the individual who wishes to practice it to reflect deeply upon the values and expectations of contemporary culture, as well as the nature of sexuality. To succeed in fulfilling this ideal one must take a wholistic approach and apply it patiently and persistently.

Greedlessness (*aparigrahaḥ)* includes not fantasizing over material possessions, nor coveting things belonging to others. Often people fantasize that if they could only become suddenly rich, by winning the lottery or marrying someone with lots of money, or winning big in the stock market, they would find lasting happiness. This is pure folly. Indulging in such fantasy simply distracts one from the inner source of lasting joy.

Tirumantiram lists ten restraints (*yama)* in verse 554:

> He does not kill, he does not lie, he does not steal,
> Of marked virtue he is; good, meek and just;
> He shares his joys, he knows no blemish;
> Neither drinks nor lusts.

The restraints (*yamas)* regulate and harmonize the *yogin*'s social life, and create the foundation for our practice. They may be difficult to observe at first, and require much conscious effort and exertion of will, but as we develop, their observance becomes not only habitual, but virtually effortless - a function of our Self-realization.

Practice: Without judging yourself or others, calmly observe your actions and feelings in relationship to others, and observe the results.

Remember the restraints (*yamas*), as a means of cultivating detachment (*vairāgya*) and discernment between the Seer and the Seen (*viveka-khyāti*). Take note of times when you forget these restraints. Cultivate affirmations to reinforce your practice of the restraints. (see verse II.33 and II,34)

31. *jāti-deśa-kāla-samaya-anavacchinnāḥ sarva-bhaumā mahā-vratam*

jāti = class

deśa = place

kāla = time

samaya = circumstance, agreement, coming together, commitment

anavacchinnāḥ = not limited by

sārva-bhaumāḥ = (from sarva-bhūmiḥ) comprising the whole world; universal

mahāvratam = great vow, resolve, conduct or decision

This Great Vow is universal, not limited by class, place, time or circumstance.

Here Patañjali affirms that these ethical principles are to be followed regardless of our status. Even the accomplished *yogin* does not have a license to ignore them. Crazy wise adepts of various spiritual traditions have at times ignored them, and as a result have brought controversy or ruin upon themselves.**(6)**

This great vow (*mahā-vratam*) greatly aids the student of *Yoga* in surmounting egoistic desires and in the attainment of surrender. In order to be totally undisturbed by whatever happens outwardly we need purity of heart. To keep equanimity and absence of reactions even the great ones must be freed of anything, which would taint their character.

Many practitioners of *Yoga* are surprised when "spiritual masters" fail to live up to the restraints (*yamas*) and observances (*niyamas*).

They fail to realize that one can have great spiritual realization and yogic accomplishments (*siddhis*) and still have a subconscious filled with negative tendencies. This is why in *Babaji's Kriya Yoga* we begin with *śuddhi dhyāna kriyā*, the first *dhyāna kriya* taught in *Babaji's Kriyā Yoga* level I initiation, to cleanse the subconscious mind. It is a long process, but even a little effort will help dispel many of the distractions. As will be seen in verses II.33 and II.34, aside from cleansing the subconscious, the student of *Yoga* will find it useful to counter-act negative thoughts with positive ones. When others, including "spiritual masters", do fail to live up to all of the *yamas* and *niyamas*, we should not condemn them. We should give them a "broom," and encourage them to clean up their basement, just as everyone else must. We must not, however, give away our power to them. Everyone is responsible for his or her own acts and failings. Furthermore, until and unless the higher consciousness has completely descended even into the vital and physical bodies and transformed them, there is always a great risk that the egoistic tendencies will resist and create problems. Constant vigilance and self-control are required to apply these first two limbs right up to the highest level of Self-realization.

Practice: Apply these restraints *(yamas)* in various situations, for example at work, in dealing with "difficult persons" or in facing temptations. Reflect upon the following: "The body is supple and impersonal, without personal will. Without any personal will, like a transmitter, let That pass through, untainted." Practice *śuddhi dhyāna kriyā* in daily life.

32. *śauca-saṃtoṣa-tapaḥ-svādhyāya-īśvara-praṇidhānāni niyamāḥ*

śauca = purity

saṃtoṣa = contentment

tapas = constant practice; intense effort; austerity

svādhyāya = self-study
īśvara-praṇidhāna = worship of God or self-surrender; surrender to the Lord

niyamāḥ = observances

Observances [*niyamas*] consist of purity, contentment, accepting but not causing pain, self-study and surrender to the Lord.

The observances [*niyamas*] are concerned with self-discipline. In verse II.1, self-study (*svādhyāya),* surrender to the Lord *(īśvara-praṇidhāna)* and constant practice (*tapas)* were discussed. Purification is to be done at the physical, vital and mental levels. Contentment (*saṁtoṣa)* can be cultivated by appreciating what we have, and desiring no more than what is necessary for maintaining one's life. The *yamas* and *niyamas* remind us of the Ten Commandments in the Judaic-Christian-Islamic traditions. We can find similar injunctions to ethical behavior in many religious traditions. However, the reward for their observance is not heaven or moral virtue, but fulfillment of a necessary pre-requisite for Self-realization.

In *Tirumantiram* verse 556, there are ten observances (*niyamas)* listed:

> Purity, compassion, frugal food and patience,
> Forthrightness, truth and steadfastness -
> These he ardently cherishes;
> Killing, stealing and lusting he abhors
> Thus stands with virtues ten
> The one who *niyama's* ways observe.

In TM verse 557 another ten attributes of *niyama* are given:

> *Tapas,* meditation, serenity and holiness
> Charity, vows in *Śaiva* way and *siddhānta* learning
> Sacrifice, *Śiva, pūja,* and thoughts pure
> With these ten, the one in *niyama* perfects His way.

There can be no physical or spiritual life without an order and rhythm. The *niyamas* are means for a harmonious and orderly life, which aids to efficiency and perfection and makes the *sādhaka (yogin)* fit for whatever work is given to him, or her.

Practice: Meditate on each of these observances using the fourth meditation *kriyā* (*arūpa dhyāna kriyā),* taught in *Babaji's Kriya Yoga* level II initiation.

33. *vitarka-bādhana pratipakṣa-bhāvanam*

vitarka = observation and analysis of material nature (see I.17); here: negative thoughts; discursive thoughts

bādhane = bondage, inhibiting

pratipakṣa = opposite

bhāvanam = cultivation; can also mean meditation

[When] bound by negative thoughts, [their] opposite [i.e. positive] ones should be cultivated. [This is] *pratipakṣa bhāvanam.*

Here "negative thoughts" include all those, which contravene the moral principles indicated by the *yamas* and *niyamas*, listed in the previous verses. Rather than indulging or rationalizing them, Patañjali prescribes direct action: the cultivation of opposite thoughts (*pratipakṣa-bhāvanam).* For example, if we feel resentment towards someone, we should develop thoughts of forgiveness. Similarly, if there is fear, thoughts of courage or confidence should be cultivated. While Patañjali does not elaborate upon the practice of *pratipakṣa bhāvanam* we know that *siddhas* like Patañjali were first-rate psychologists. To counter deep-seated tendencies towards negative thinking required regular and diligent practice of such things as affirmations, autosuggestion and self-hypnosis. The subconscious mind, not unlike a computer, continues to operate according to suggestions which are programmed into it since early childhood even when they are harmful or cause suffering. Such suggestions come from our parents, our friends, our teachers, the mass media and the cultural symbols and values, which permeate our world. In the contemporary field of Yoga it is a wonder that our teachers and authorities have for the most part failed to emphasize or teach the scientific art of autosuggestion and affirmation. Too often, those who enter a spiritual lifestyle assume that their spiritual practices will automatically heal deep-seated psychological conflicts. While psychotherapy may initially help, it often lacks a wider spiritual perspective. Ultimately the healing process requires each person to skillfully counter all unwholesome thoughts and emotions without merely suppressing them. (See reference 7 for practical techniques to implement this verse)

Practice: Identify and categorize habitual negative thinking. Cultivate affirmations and auto-suggestions to skillfully counter these negative tendencies. Meditate on the positive feelings associated with the positive suggestions or affirmations you create. Practice forgiveness.

34. *vitarkā hiṃsā-ādayaḥ kṛta-kārita-anumoditā lobha-krodha-moha-pūrvakā mṛdu-madhya-adhimātrā duḥkha-ajñāna-ananta-phalā iti pratipakṣa-bhāvanam*

vitarkāḥ = here: negative thoughts; discursive thoughts

hiṁsā-ādayaḥ = violence, etc.

kṛta = done

kārita = caused to be done

anumoditāḥ = approved; permitted

lobha = greed; lust

krodha = anger, passion

moha = infatuation; delusion

pūrvakāḥ = preceded by, accompanied by

mṛdu = mild

madhya = medium; moderate

adhimātrāḥ = intense
duḥkha = pain; dissatisfaction

ajñāna = ignorance

ananta = infinite; boundless; eternal

phalā = fruits; resultants

iti = thus

pratipakṣa = opposite thoughts, literally "the opposite side" or "an opponent or foe"

bhāvanam = meditation; producing, manifesting; cultivating

When negative thoughts or acts such as violence, etc. are caused to be done or even approved of, whether incited by greed, anger or infatuation, whether indulged in with mild, moderate or extreme intensity, they are based on ignorance and bring certain pain. [Hence] Opposite thoughts should be cultivated.

Patañjali makes very clear the consequences of indulging negative thought, in whatever form or degree, and the importance of cultivating their opposites. The *yogin* is to be circumspect about negative thoughts and not indulge them even in a mild way. This recalls verse II.1 where he defines *Kriyā Yoga* as self-study (*svādhyāya*). The practice of recording what passes through one's mind, when done with detachment (*vairāgya*), can indicate to each individual what needs to be countered. Modern techniques of self-hypnosis and affirmations can then be applied (see reference 7).

Sometimes we must remove ourselves physically from a situation, or atmosphere, where negative thinking prevails. If that is not possible, then consider the difficulties as opportunities to cultivate equanimity and detachment from negative reactions. Pray and seek Divine support and guidance. Meditate with a focus on the heart concentrated on the feeling of love. When negative thoughts arise, jot them down and note what emotion brought them up. Awareness is the first step.

Practice: Keep a journal, and note your negative tendencies. Apply methods of autosuggestion and affirmation to cultivate their opposite.

35. *ahiṃsā-pratiṣṭhāyāṃ tat-saṃnidhau vaira-tyāgaḥ*

ahiṃsā = non-violence

pratiṣṭhāyam = having established

tat = that

saṃnidhau = presence, nearness

vaira = hostility

tyāgaḥ = given up; abandonment

In the presence of one firmly established in non-violence, all hostilities cease.

By cultivating peace within, the *yogin* creates a space where all may find peace. Our thoughts affect others, usually negatively; hence the average person finds peace usually alone, or in nature. The *yogin's* state of mind is a great gift to the world. He or she can help to heal everyone around them. If adversity comes, such a *yogin* welcomes it as an opportunity to heal it. They are truly the hope for this world with all of its hostilities and suffering.

In India there are many stories of saints who, living in the forest were not disturbed by wild animals. The influence of Mahatma Gandhi, who started the non-violence movement for political emancipation of India, continues today in movements for civil rights and others.

According to the Mother of the Sri Aurobindo Ashram, pure existence *(sat)* is, outside of manifestation. It is wonderfully luminous, immobile, tranquil, and a bliss devoid of vibration. It is very useful. We should keep it in the background of consciousness and refer to it to correct all disturbances. Keep it there all the time as if supporting everything from behind. It is by nature silent, immobile and luminous, and it gives the sense of Eternity and Infinity. It is the cure for disorder.

Practice: Reflect upon *sat,* pure beingness, luminous, silent, tranquil and blissful. Remember it in relating to everything.

36. *satya-pratiṣṭhāyāṃ kriyā-phala-āśrayatvam*

satya = truthfulness

pratiṣṭhāyām = having established

kriyā = action

phala = fruits or results

āśrayatvam = depend upon; correspondence; depending on; following

To one established in truthfulness, actions and their results depend upon [him].

Literally, this means that if a person is always truthful, a time will come when all that he says will come true. The *yogīn* gets the power to attract whatever he seeks automatically. Nature provides. However, when we indulge in fantasy or half-truths, we dissipate our energy. The forces of the universe cannot easily flow through us unless we remain centered in truth and Self-realization.

One established in truthfulness *(satya)* becomes fearless, as there is nothing to hide. Truthfulness requires effort at first, because we are in the habit of lying, especially to ourselves, but with practice it will become easy, especially when we notice the wonderful effects of being honest.

Practice: Reflect upon: "Am I able to look at everything in my life without distortion? Am I willing to see what is really in front of me, instead of what I want to see?"

37. *asteya-pratiṣṭhāyāṃ sarva-ratna-upasthānam*

asteya = non-stealing

pratiṣṭhāyam = [having] established

sarva = all
ratna = gem, jewel; wealth, riches

upasthānam = presence, appearance

Wealth comes to all established in non-stealing.

Along the same lines as II.36 this means that when the *yogīn* is established in non-stealing, wealth comes to him. Stealing occurs when we desire something that does not belong to us, and then one acts upon that desire. In a broader sense, it also involves greed, fantasizing about what we lack, and even if we have wealth, it involves hoarding it. Patañjali reminds us that like a current of water, nature seeks to flow through us; when we become greedy or hoard things, she directs her bounty elsewhere. Put even more simply, "it's better to give than to receive." For when we give we allow the universe to give us more, and to work through us. Ultimately we realize, like the *karma yogin*, that we are not the doer; we cease to take credit for things accomplished - we cease to misappropriate, or steal the credit.

If we are established in non-stealing, we strive to do the work, or to work things out with a lot of care, without tension, without expectation of a return. All wealth comes with selflessness. We are awarded with the four things that make us truly wealthy: equality, peace, spiritual ease in all circumstances and joy and laughter of the soul.

Practice: Reflect on this: Am I able to give without wanting something in return?

38. *brahmacarya-pratiṣṭhāyāṃ vīrya-lābhaḥ*

brahmacarya = chastity; sexual restraint

pratiṣṭhāyām = having established

vīrya = vigor; power, strength, energy

lābha = gained; obtained

By one established in chastity, vigor is gained.

Chastity (*brahmacarya),* is detachment from sexual fantasies. Fantasizing about sex, or indulging lustful feelings, dissipates and disperses the mind just as the physical acts of sex cause the loss of vital force. The cultivation of *brahmacarya* enables us to sublimate vital energy to awaken the higher centers of consciousness, and to turn the consciousness away from fleeting sense sensations and towards the ultimate inner source of joy.

Even in marriage we should practice moderation with regard to sexual activity, and seek to transmute sexual energies through both practices and attitudes. We may see our spouse as a living embodiment of the Divine.

In *Tirumantiram* verse 1938:

> He to lust a slave becomes,
> Will in constant fear be;
> His body deteriorates,
> And his life ebbs away
> He will not Grace receive
> And in *Śiva Yoga* lasts not.

In verses 1952:

> In ignorance the folks waste it daily;
> And destroyed by senses, in pain weep;
> If in wisdom, they conscious perform *Yoga* supreme,
> The *bindu* (transmuted spiritual energy) disappears, divinely assimilated.

By going above ourselves we can get out of problems, but the problems below are still there and need to be resolved. By going deep within to the emotional being and opening the heart-center to peace and untroubled aspiration for the Divine, chastity becomes effortless.

But, as Sri Aurobindo puts it: when we cling to the "Thou Shalts" and the "Thou Shalt nots," what is harmful for one person may be helpful for another.**(8)** What may be harmful under certain circumstances may be helpful in other conditions. What is done in a certain spirit may be disastrous, yet the same thing done in a quite different spirit would be innocuous, or even beneficial. There are many things to be considered: the spirit, the circumstances, the person, the need and the cast of the nature, the stage. That is why it is said that the *guru* must deal with each disciple according to his separate nature and accordingly guide his *sādhana*; even if it is the same line of sadhana for all, yet at every point for each it differs.

Practice: Am I able to keep God in my heart, mind and body when I am having a sexual experience? Am I able to make love as an offering to the Divine. Am I able to remain as the Seer in relation with the Seen? Am I able to see my partner as an embodiment of the Divine?

39. *aparigraha-sthairye janma-kathaṃtā-saṃbodhaḥ*

aparigraha = greedlessness

sthairye = settled, being established in; in firmness, stability or steadfastness

janma-kathaṃtā = the "how and why" of birth

saṃbodha = illuminated knowledge; understanding

When one is established in greedlessness, illuminated knowledge of the how and why of one's birth comes.

As we give up greed *(aparigraha)* or attachment, we begin to identify more and more with the Self. From the Self's perspective, which ranges beyond time and place, knowledge of previous births and tendencies becomes accessible. We are no longer tied down to the limited current set of ego-based desires. The storehouse of deep-seated habitual tendencies in the subconscious becomes accessible. It is important to see them with detachment. Many who do not, become overwhelmed by such memories.

When the wanting for our individual selves is finally released and we surrender our preferences, remembering, "Let Thy will be done," then greedlessness is established. We begin to work at deeper and deeper levels. Sometimes when a subconscious impression (*saṁskāra)* is about to come to the surface to be released, knowledge of a past life experience, which precipitated the *saṁskāra,* will also surface. Perhaps this is so that the limitation or tendency can be totally and finally eradicated from the body-mind. It is best not to get too interested or involved in the revelation, but simply to "allow" the release which comes from it and which prepares the body to make it more receptive for change.

Practice: Reflect upon the question: "Am I willing to let everything go? Also "Let Thy will be done."

40. *śaucāt-sva-aṅga-jugupsā parair-asaṃsargaḥ*

> *śauca* = purity
>
> *sva-aṅga* = one's own body
>
> *jugupsā* = spontaneous detachment
>
> *paraiḥ* = with others
>
> *asaṁsarga* = no contact or no association.

By purification arises spontaneous detachment for one's own body and no contact with other [bodies].

In the context of the present verse *(jugupsā)* may also imply something more positive or balanced; that is detachment or wariness towards one's own body and its contact with others. Knowing the difficulty of the path to Self-realization and being aware of the tendencies of the mind to indulge thoughts of lust, for example, the *yogin* seeks to minimize the risk of failure by avoiding contact with other bodies.

The physical body is constantly processing waste materials, particularly through the skin. Most persons attempt to mask this using clothing, deodorants, perfumes and cosmetics. Probably more than 90 percent of our waking hours is devoted to taking care of the physical body directly or indirectly. Eventually, however, the *yogin's* disgust may mature into a new perspective. The *yogin* may see his body in a better way. As Tirumūlar says in TM verse 725:

> Time was when I despised the body;
> But then I saw the God within
> And the Body I realized, is the Lord's temple
> And so I began preserving it

With care infinite.

Practice: Reflect on the question: "Am I the physical body?"

41. *sattva-śuddhi-saumanasya-eka-agrya-indriya-jaya-ātma-darśana-yogyatvāni ca*

sattvaśuddhi = purity of being

saumanasya = gladness of mind, cheerfulness

ekagrya = one-pointedness

indriyajaya = mastery of the five senses

ātmadarśana = realization or correct vision of the Self

yogyatvāni = fitness, suitability

ca = and

Moreover one gains purity of being, joy in the mind, one pointedness, mastery over the senses and fitness for Self-realization.

There is no single English word, which can translate *sattva*. It is the constituent force of Nature which brings equilibrium; the mode of peace, balance, poise and brightness. Literally, it means "beingness." As a result of going through the process of purification (see verses I.2 and II.28, 29 and 30) one develops it, as well as mental joy, or delight, which is independent of outer circumstances; the mind easily focuses and ceases to be distracted either by desires or sensory input. Finally, it brings the capacity for Self -realization. By following the *yamas* and *niyamas* we gain this purity of being *(śuddhisattva)*, the first of the five observances (*niyama)*.

Practice: Meditate on the purity of being *(śuddhisattva)*.

42. *saṃtosād-anuttamaḥ sukha-lābhaḥ*

saṃtosād = because of or from contentment

anuttamaḥ = supreme; unsurpassed, excellent

sukha = joy, happiness

lābhaḥ = gained, obtained

By contentment, supreme joy is gained.

Contentment *(saṁtoṣaḥ),* (see verse II.32) one of the observances *(niyamas)* involves neither liking nor disliking; it occurs when one is simply being oneself. The nature of our being is absolute joy *(ānanda).* There is nothing to do, but to appreciate it, or observe it.

Contentment is an inner poise, which implies harmony, delight in oneself and inner love, wherein one is untroubled by difficulties around oneself. Whether anyone feels it, or not, is due to his or her openness to it.

Practice: Share your contentment and joy with others, but not your discontent. Practice seeing the best in others, not their faults.

43. *kāya-indriya-siddhir-aṣuddhi-kṣayāt-tapasaḥ*

kāya = body

indriya = sense organ

siddhi = perfection, attainment; accomplishment

aṣuddhi = impurity

kṣayāt = due to destruction

tapasaḥ = because of austerity; constant practice

By austerity, impurities of the body and senses are destroyed and perfection gained.

By constant practice *(tapas),* or sustained effort, impurity (aś*uddhi*) which limit the physical, vital and mental are gradually eliminated.

As a result the five subtle senses corresponding to the physical senses (such as clairvoyance, seeing without the eyes, clairaudience, hearing without the ears, etc.) develop and the body becomes invulnerable, graceful and beautiful (see verse III.46 for an elaboration of perfection of the body or *kāya-siddhi*). In *Tirumantiram* there are more than a hundred different references to the perfection of the body and the sense(s) *(kāya indriya siddhiḥ)*.

For example:

> Having abated not in the rules of vows
> The *Yogin* who has to meditate learned
> Coursing *kuṇḍalini* through the spinal column
> And passing *maṇḍalas* three with felicity equal
> He in fleshy body forever lives. (TM 612)
>
> If the body perishes, *prāṇa* departs
> Nor will the Light of Truth be reached
> I learned the way of preserving my body
> And so doing, my *prāṇa* too. (TM724)
>
> If the seminal seed thickens by sexual abstention,
> It (the body) shall never be destroyed
> If the body is lightened by austere discipline
> Long shall the life be;
> If food is taken sparingly
> Many the good that flow;
> You may verily become
> The Lord of Dark hued throat (*Śiva* with a blue throat or *Nīlakaṇṭha*) (TM 735)

"One must not treat the human nature like a machine to be handled according to rigid mental rules; a great plasticity is needed in dealing with its complex motives." Sri Aurobindo. However, he adds, there must be a control over the emotions and the ego in order for there to be harmony and unity in the body and in life itself. Of course, in *Yoga,* where we speak of ridding ourselves of the ego and rising to states of perfection, strict rules of conduct and discipline are expedient. Personal discretion within a certain framework is allowed, as long as it is discreetly used. In *Yoga,* ultimately, it is obedience to the *guru*, or the Divine, or the law of Truth, which is the foundation of a spiritual life. What may look as an austerity to some may simply be consciously making the right choices.

Practice: Reflect on these questions: "What in your daily life might others consider as an austerity?" "Do you consider it an austerity or simply a way of life?"

44. *svādhyāyād-iṣṭa-devatā-saṃprayogaḥ*

svādhyāyāt = from or because of self-study

iṣṭadevatā = chosen deity

saṃprayoga = communion

By self-study [comes] communion with one's chosen deity.

Self study *(svādhyāya)* was presented in verse II.1 as one of the three principal means of Patañjali's *Kriyā Yoga*, along with constant repeated practice (*tapas)* and surrender to the Lord (*Īśvara-praṇidhāna*). Here, he indicates that self-study enables one to draw closer to our chosen form of God *(iṣṭa-devatā).* How so? As explained in the commentary on verse II.1, becoming aware of what we are not, makes us increasingly aware of what we truly are: *Īsvara.* The study of sacred texts may also remind us of Who we truly are. In the beginning we may find it easier to project our love for the Divine on something external to ourselves, and it is certainly easier to focus on a form, rather than the formless; hence the popularity of a great variety of images, or forms of God. The one we are most attracted to is known as our *iṣṭa-devatā*, or chosen deity. But as discussed in the introduction, the *siddhas* were distinguished by an absence of any such worship of deities. The *siddhas* discovered that inside themselves lay the Supreme Lord.

Some have argued that the Classical *Yoga* of Patañjali excludes the possibility of Union (*saṁyoga*) between one's Self and *Īsvara,* or the Lord.**(9)** This may be true if one assumes Patañjali was a strict adherent of Sa*ṁkhyā* philosophy, which is dualistic and in its early form, even denies the existence of a Supreme Being. However, in verses such as this and the next one, as well as verse I.23, Patañjali clearly indicates our potential for communion with the Lord. In the introduction of this volume, I have stated that Patañjali shared Tirumūlar's and the Tamil *siddhas* philosophy and theology. While all of them used language, which denoted dualism, this referred only to the bound or deluded condition of the average person, prior to Self-realization. Our soul's communion *(saṁyoga)* with our chosen deity (*iṣṭa-devatā)* would mean, "they are not two," and that the "*jīva* is becoming *Śiva.*" Bound souls, ignorant of their true nature, become liberated and commune with their Lord once they, through self-study, distinguish their true Self from the personality and mental movements. This is even clearer in the next verse.

When we begin to deeply study our selves, we begin to discover within our own hearts, qualities that not only are attributes of our favorite conception of the Supreme Being *(iṣṭa-devatā)*, but are also attributes of our inner Self. Everything has the same constituent elements, and so every change lies in the interrelationship of things. If there is but one power, one substance, one consciousness, one truth, then the only thing we lack is awareness of that Oneness. Communion *(saṁprayogaḥ)* comes slowly with that awareness. Communion comes in all flavors. We may hear, see, taste, feel or know. Communion may be awakened in a way which is so subtle that we are unaware, but it is there. It gently leads us, informs us, comforts us, and even carries us at times.

Practice: Reflect on this: The most important thing for the purification of the heart is absolute sincerity and honesty with God-*Guru*-Self. Communicate with That without pretense, without concealment, and without lies or distortions of the truth. Confession helps to purge the consciousness of hampering elements and it clears the inner air and makes for a more intimate relationship to God-*Guru*-Self. As Jesus said: "The Truth shall set you free."

45. *samādhi-siddhir-īśvara-praṇidhānāt*

samādhi = cognitive absorption

siddhir = attainment, power
īśvara-praṇidhānāt = because of or from surrender or devotion to the Lord

Because of [one's] surrender to the Lord, cognitive absorption is attained.

Here Patañjali elaborates on the fifth observance (*niyama*), that is "surrender" or devotion to the Lord (*īśvara-praṇidhāna*). While it is the only one of the observances which is specifically related to cognitive absorption (*samādhi)*, there is nothing to indicate that the other four *niyamas*, which are, purity (*śuddhi*), contentment *(saumanasya)*, constant practice (*tapas)* and self study (*svādhyāya)*, are any less important or that devotion to the Lord *(īśvara-praṇidhāna)* is an alternative to them. Like a cake recipe, these five *niyamas* go together and their combination is synergistic. Surrender to the Lord was earlier described in I.23 as a means to *samādhi.* As discussed in verse II.1, Patañjali defines the three main practices of his *Kriyā Yoga* as surrender to the Lord, self study and constant practice, aside from the practice of detachment *(vairāgya).*

While surrender to the Lord implies a state of duality between the devotee and the Beloved, the attainment (*siddhi*) of cognitive absorption (*samādhi)* involves going beyond duality into non-duality or unity.

Like Patañjali, Tirumūlar expresses this going beyond separateness into oneness by means of devotion:

> He is Our Own
> He is the Primal One
> He taught the *Vedas* Four
> He is the light that glows within the purest gold
> They adored Him in Love
> They approached Him all desires devoid
> All climbed the Mystic Tree High
> Their breath halted in *Samādhi*
> They with him became One. (TM 626)

In TM 136:

> The fierce rays of the sun beating upon the water
> The dissolved salt does in crystal shapes emerge;
> That salt in the water dissolved becomes liquid again,
> So does *Jīva* in *Śiva* get redissolved.

While the salt and the water are different, "they are not two."

One opens to the Lord and sooner or later one is absorbed in the Lord. One meditates on the Lord, and the qualities of the same. We must not be impatient. The Lord Himself is doing everything at the time He chooses. When we accept with gratitude that He is doing everything, and that there is nothing for us to do, not even yearn for, then it comes. It is simple and spontaneous and all we have to do is to surrender to the Lord with all our heart and body and mind.

Practice: Think of the Lord always, in whatever way you feel drawn to.

46. *sthira-sukham-āsanam*

sthira = steady

sukha = comfortable

āsanam = posture

***Āsana* is a steady, comfortable posture.**

Here Patañjali indicates what characterizes a *Yoga* posture (*āsana*). It must enable the practitioner to remain steady: that is, immobile and it must be comfortable: that is enable one to relax. Later in the medieval period, around the 12th'century, *Haṭha Yoga* was further developed as a means to gain mastery over physical and subtle energetic processes, leading to the awakening of the kundalini energy. Nowhere in the Sutras do we find any references to *kuṇḍalini,* subtle energy centres (*cakras)* or psychic channels (*naḍīs),* so dear to the *Haṭha yogin* or *yoga tantrika.* This does not mean that they were unknown to Patañjali, but that he simply chose not to include them. In *Tirumantiram* 558-563, eight important postures (*āsanas),* all of which fulfill Patañjali's requirements for steadiness and comfort, are described in detail. This is probably the oldest written description of *Yoga āsanas.* Tirumūlar goes on to mention 180 other important postures (*āsanas)* without naming them:

Bhadra, Gomukha, Padma and *Siṁha*
Sothira, Vīra, and Sukha

These seven along with eminent *Svāstika*
Constitute the eight. Eighty and hundred however
Are *āsanas* in all reckoned. (TM 563)

In contemporary schools of *Yoga*, this emphasis on relaxation, comfort and steadiness is often lost, as *Yoga* becomes combined with such things as aerobics and dance, and the emphasis shifts to performance of ever more difficult postures. When divorced from its purpose, postures (*āsanas*) serve the values of contemporary culture: looking good, competition and individualism.

Practice: Practice *Babaji's Kriyā Haṭha Yoga* in stages and pairs, with relaxation periods in between.

47. *prayatna-śaithilya-ananta-samāpattibhyām*

prayatna = effort, striving, exertion; tension

śaithilya = relaxation, looseness

ananta = infinite

samāpattibhyām = [two kinds of] cognitive absorption, balanced state[s]

From the relaxation of tension and endless unity [*samadhi* is established].

When a posture (*āsana*) is done correctly, not only will it be steady and comfortable, but also all tension (*prayatna*), both physical and mental, will subside, and ultimately the breathless state of cognitive absorption (*samādhi*) will ensue. This process is described in verse I.41. The body feels like pure sensation, pure vibration. The Psalmist's words remind us of the ultimate purpose of a *Yoga āsana* correctly performed:

"Be Still, and Know That I am God."

Practice: Select one posture (*āsana*) and master it. To master a posture it must become effortless. One can remain in it with ease for an indefinite length of time, to the point where we can meditate in it. Allow the support of a pillow or blanket as needed.

48. *tato dvandva-anabhighātāḥ*

tato = thereafter; thus, from that

dvandva = dualities; a pair of opposites

anabhighātāḥ = invulnerable

Thereafter one is invulnerable to the dualities.

When a *Yoga āsana* is steady and comfortable and induces a state of deep relaxation and cognitive absorption, the consciousness is withdrawn from the external world with all of its dualities *(dvandvas).* We become oblivious to whether it is hot or cold, or whether pain is absent or present in the body.

There may be a feeling of a pleasant numbness, or a spontaneous *āsana* may occur. There may be a sense of going into deeper depths.

Practice: Once you have mastered a posture, use it frequently for meditation. You may experience profound peace in the *āsana,* or a calm, which is merely an absence of disturbance in the body, or you may feel a certain stability and strength arising from the calm.

49. *tasmin-sati śvāsa-praśvāsayor-gati-vicchedaḥ prāṇāyāmaḥ*

tasmin = in this or that

sati = being

śvāsa = inhalation; breath

praśvāsayor = of the exhalations

gati = motion, origin, scope, condition

vicchedaḥ = cutting off, breaking; separating, interrupting; cessation; here: control

prāṇāyāma = breath control

With regard to [these postures] breath control is the control of the motions of inhalation and exhalation.

While the term *vicchedaḥ* (see II.4) literally means, "cutting off" in the context of breathing it means "controlling, or regulating, the inhalation and the exhalation." This includes controlling the space between, that is the possible period of retention, because of its effect upon the mental movements (see I.34).

Practice: As you bring the body to stillness, draw the breath into it, being conscious of the inhalation and exhalation. Use the breath to still the body, allow it to become and remain, firm and comfortable. Use the breath to sink deeper into the posture.

50. *bāhya-abhyantara-stambha-vṛttir-deśa-kāla-saṃkhyābhiḥ paridṛṣṭo dīrgha-sūkṣmaḥ*

bāhya = external, outer

abhyantara = internal, inside

stambha = stationary, suppressed, stopped

vṛttir = fluctuation

deśa = place; space

kāla = time

saṃkhyābhiḥ = by or with observation or calculation, number

paridṛṣṭa = seen, beheld, perceived

dīrgha = long, lofty, tall

sūkṣma = subtle

Breath control is external, internal or stationary. It is perceived according to time, space and number and [becomes long and subtle]

There are three phases to breath control *(prāṇāyāma)*: inhalation (internal or *abhyantara*), exhalation (external or *bāhya*) or retention (fixed or *stambha*). Furthermore, it can include directing the flow of the breath mentally to a particular place (*desa*) in the body, for example, towards a particular subtle energy centre or wheel in the body (*cakra*). Time (*kāla*) should also be regulated, by counting the length of the breath. The number of repetitions or count (*saṁkhyaḥ*) needs to be controlled. This is because if done excessively or incorrectly, *prāṇāyāma* can lead to unpleasant reactions. It should therefore be learned from one who is experienced in its practice and who can guide the student through potential difficulties. There are many different types of *prāṇāyāma*, each with their own effects.

Practice: Direct the exhalation mentally into the heat, or discomfort, in the posture. Think of the breath as softening the body, not forcing it. You are mastering the posture when your breath is relaxed and flowing and silence begins to descend. Learn and practice the various *prāṇyāmas* in *Babaji's Kriyā Yoga*, especially *kriyā kuṇḍalini prāṇāyāma*.

51. *bāhya-abhyantara-viṣaya-ākṣepī caturthaḥ*

bāhya = external

abhyantara = internal

viṣaya = condition; object

ākṣepī = withdrawal

caturtha = the fourth

There is a fourth during withdrawal [between] internal and external conditions [of breathing].

Here Patañjali refers to a particular practice (well known to advanced students of *Babaji's Kriya Yoga*) wherein we focus upon an object of concentration between the inhalation and exhalation. As the breathing slows, this interval grows, and as the concentration on this object deepens, the breathing slows even more until eventually the breathing and the mind become still and we enter into a state of cognitive absorption (*samādhi*). This particular practice is generally preceded by other forms of *prāṇāyāma*, as described in verse 49 and 50.

Practice: Practice the *haṁsa* (literally "swan") meditation, while following the breath.

52. *tataḥ kṣīyate prakāśa-āvaraṇam*

tataḥ = as a result; then

kṣīyate = is destroyed; is dissolved; diminished

prakāśa = light; brightness; splendor

āvaraṇam = veil; concealment; covering

As a result, the veil over [the inner] Light is destroyed.

Here Patañjali refers to a particular state: "the falling of the veil around the inner light" (familiar to advanced students of *Babaji's Kriya Yoga*). In the same way as a veil may be removed, thread by thread, *prāṇāyāma* has the effect of removing, one by one, the thoughts which in their totality create an inner darkness. What is revealed is the underlying Light of consciousness. Until then we are like a child, who when it looks at a wooden horse, sees only a horse, and not the wood.

Practice: Persist in physical *sādhana*. *Haṭha Yoga* opens the body to energy and joy and deep peace and relaxation.

53. *dhāraṇāsu ca yogyatā manasaḥ*

dhāraṇāsu = in, concerning concentration

ca = and

yogyatā = fitness

manasaḥ = of the mind

And the mind becomes fit for concentration.

The gradual removal of the inner veil (*āvaraṇam)* of mental darkness facilitates the practice of concentration (*dhārāṇā*). So the experience of the inner light (*prakaśa)* is not an end in itself. As the body, mind and breath relaxes and the inner Light is revealed, natural resistance will begin to fall away. Concentration becomes simple as the mind, body and breath become calm.

Practice: Be at ease; allow life to be simple (especially when it feels "complicated").

54. *sva-viṣaya-asaṃprayoge cittasya sva-rūpa-anukāra iva-indriyāṇāṃ pratyāhāraḥ*

sva = own

viṣaya = circumstance; condition; object

asaṃprayoge = disengagement; disunite

cittasya = of mind; of consciousness

svarūpa = one's own form

anukāra = imitation, resemblance,

iva = as if, just as

indriyāyāṇaṁ = of the sense organs
pratyāhāra = withdrawal

When the senses disunite themselves from their own objects and resemble, as it were, their own form of consciousness, this is sense withdrawal.

Prāṇāyāma is not sufficient in itself to control the restless mind, because of the activity of the senses (*indriyāḥ*). When the five senses of seeing, hearing, tasting, touching and smelling are active, consciousness unites with the sense objects and in effect we forget our Self. For example, if one feels hot, one says, "I am hot." However, when we restrict the action of the five senses, for example, by closing the eyes and sitting comfortably with no distractions, consciousness ceases to identify with external sense objects, and the five senses become like consciousness itself: formless, calm and centered inwardly. The senses are like a mirror: when they are turned outside, they reflect the world of forms; turned inwards, they reflect the pure formless light. We must assume the forms of what the senses allow in. If we frequently look at pictures of saints and divine beings, our mind assumes their form. If we frequently look at pornography or violent movies, the mind becomes lustful and violent tendencies plague us. So withdrawal (*pratyāhāra*) is control of the senses in order to control the mind. It requires discrimination in daily life, not just while sitting in meditation. Years of practice are needed to master it. We may cultivate it by choosing leisure activities, which will uplift our consciousness and remind ourselves of our highest ideals. Even food should be eaten as an offering to the Divine (*prasāda*). Swami Ramdas observed his chosen deity (*iṣṭa devatā*) "*Rāma*" in everything and everyone and accepted all events as the will of Rāma. This is a higher form of sense withdrawal (*pratyāhāra*).

When the light and the peace are felt within us, it will remain as a basis for right actions in our whole nature. We will remain undisturbed and not pulled outward or invaded by anything our senses become aware of.

Practice: Consider what you are allowing to invade your consciousness. Move away from things, which are disturbing to your peace of mind. What is important in your discrimination is whether or not your inner connection with the Self remains.

55. *tataḥ paramā vaśyatā-indriyāṇām*

tata = thence; then

paramā = supreme

vaśyatā = mastery

indriya = sense

Then [you should have] supreme mastery over the senses.

In this last verse of the second chapter, which deals with *sādhāna*, the path to realization, Patañjali does not elaborate upon what supreme mastery of the senses gives, but we can infer that by its position at the end of the chapter, that it is the springboard to the next chapter which deals with the accomplishments *(siddhis)*.

As we withdraw from the disturbances of the outer world our inner world becomes tranquil and our nature purer. We begin to see things as they are and not as we want them to be. We become like children in our innocence and spontaneity. We want for nothing; we are content with everything just as it is.

Tirumantiram contains ten verses on the subject of withdrawal (*pratyāhāra)*, beginning with verse 578:

> Step by step practice mind's withdrawal
> And look inward;
> One by one many the good you see within;
> And may you then meet the Lord,
> Now and here below
> Whom the ancient *Veda* still searches everywhere.

In subsequent verses he mentions that centering ones concentration in the body at various centers will enable the awakening of *kuṇḍalini*, and various experiences leading to union with the Lord.

In the last verse dealing with sense withdrawal (*pratyāhāra)*, or sense withdrawal, *Tirumantiram* states:

> In the act of *pratyāhāra*
> All the world will be visioned;
> Be rid of the despicable darkness
> And seek the Lord,

If your thoughts be centered firm,
You shall the Divine Light see
And immortal thereafter be. (TM 587)

This enriches both our understanding of how to practice it and what results may be anticipated.

Practice: In meditation, and throughout the day, practice wanting nothing, being content with everything just as it is.

Chapter 3: VIBHŪTI PĀDA

While *vibhūti* is nowhere described in the *Sūtras*, it refers to the extraordinary powers described in this chapter. In the *Tirumantiram*, *vibhūti* refers to the holy ash smeared on the body, especially upon the forehead by *Śiva yogins* (TM verse 1655-1667). This ash is the residue of the fire ceremonies *(yajñās)*, which Śaivite ascetics (*sādhus*) regularly conduct. It represents the residue of their austerities, and symbolizes the purification through the fire of intense practice (*tapas*) (see II.1) to which they subject themselves. These super human powers express the divinity, which is at the core of each individual; once the superficial ego bound layers of personality are burned away by the fire of intense practice. While Patañjali does not define *vibhūti*, we may understand it to mean, "ultimate result of intense yogic practice." Such powers are not valued for themselves, and if one becomes attached to them, they may become an obstacle to Self-realization. The term *vibhūti* is therefore an apt term, referring to both the purity resulting from constant practice and detachment from all results.

1. *deśa-bandhaś-cittasya dhāraṇā*

deśa = a place

bandhaḥ = binding

cittasya = of consciousness

dhāraṇā = concentration

Concentration is the binding of consciousness to one place, object or idea.

Concentration *(dhāraṇā)* is the fifth member of the eight limbed system of *aṣṭāṅga Yoga*. It includes all those techniques, which involve fixing the mind on a single sense object or point. It may involve the subtle senses of seeing, hearing, smelling, touching or tasting. It does not involve the physical senses such as candle gazing (a form of *trāṭaka)* or listening to music. As a result, the mind becomes steady. As stated in *Tirumantiram* verse 597:

> To contain body's harassing senses five
> In elements five,
> To contain elements five,
> In organs cognitive internal,
> To contain organs cognitive internal,
> In their *Tanmātras* (five senses)
> To contain the *tanmātras*
> In the Being uncreated,
> That verily is *Dhāraṇā*
> In stages practiced.

Initiates of *Babaji's Kriya Yoga* are taught how to concentrate on each of the five subtle sense faculties (*jñāna indriyas*), and distinguish them from the five physical senses (i.e. seeing, hearing, tasting, touching, smelling) and the five elements or *pañca-bhūta* (ether, air, fire, water and earth in which they function respectively) in a series of progressive initiations. In doing so, they become aware of the grosser realities (*tattvas)* of nature. Ultimately they learn how to free the consciousness from involvement with them.

Practice: Practice the second (single form or *eka rūpa Tam.)*, third (moving form or *īnai rūpa)* and fifth (*pūrṇa bhāva,* literally "emotion-filled"*) dhyāna kriyās,* or the concentration on material objects (*trāṭaka kriyās*).

2. *tatra pratyaya-ekatānatā dhyānam*

tatra = therein

pratyaya = intention; thought, notion, experience, belief, knowledge, basis, religious contemplation, mean

ekatānatā = having the quality of ['*tā*'] of stretching [*tāna*]; the quality of having the mind fixed on one object only

dhyānam = meditation

In this context, meditation is the experience of having the mind fixed on one object only.

Concentration (*dhāraṇā*) requires effort because the mind is continuously wandering, so one must detach from the distractions and return to the chosen object, with patience and firmness. It is easy to give up and say, "I'm not fit for meditation." By being as patient with the mind's tendencies as you would with a puppy dog that you are attempting to train, one may succeed. When concentration (*dhāraṇā*) becomes effortless, meditation (*dhyāna*) begins. That is, meditation is born out of the mastery of concentration. The object of meditation may become dynamic or involve related ideas or stories; it may be with or without form. We can define meditation as "being continually aware of a chosen object or subject." All schools of meditation could share this definition because in all schools the meditator attempt to keep continuous awareness flowing towards a chosen object or subject. What varies between different schools is the object or subject chosen: some choose the breath, or nose tip, others choose an object in nature like a rose; others choose a geometric form like a *yantra* or *maṇḍala* focused upon to invoke the deity; others choose an abstract idea, like "love;" still others practice it with eyes open on an object like a bow and arrow.

In meditation (*dhyāna*), there is, however, the object, the subject (one who meditates) and their relationship. That is, the meditator remains aware of the object and the ideas related to it. *Tirumantiram* verses 598 to 617 describes various types of meditation.

Meditation (*dhyāna*) is the scientific art of mastering the mind. It is a science because it contains all of the elements of the scientific method. It starts with a hypothesis to be tested, that is, the technique. Then there is the experiment itself, one practices the techniques. Then one records one's experiences, just as scientists do. Then one compares one's experiences with those of other practitioners or one's teacher, just as scientists do in their conferences. It is an art because it requires much practice and skill. It is not sufficient to simply have the knowledge of how to practice the technique. If that were the case, simply reading a book or attending a course in which the technique was explained could enlighten someone.

<u>Practice</u>: Practice various forms of meditation (*dhyāna*) in order to

master the mind at all levels. The mind includes the subconscious, the five physical senses and their subtle counterparts, the intellect, the psychic and the superconscious levels.

3. *tad-eva-artha-mātra-nirbhāsaṃ sva-rūpa-śūnya-iva samādhiḥ*

tad = that [meditation (*dhyāna)*]

eva = indeed

arthamātra = the whole sense or object

nirbhāsaṁ = to shine forth, to seem to be

svarūpa = own form

śūnyaṁ = empty, void

iva = as if

samādhiḥ = cognitive absorption

Cognitive absorption [*samādhiḥ*] is that meditation [when] the whole object [i.e.consciousness] shines forth, as if devoid of its own form.

In cognitive absorption (*samādhiḥ)*, meditation (*dhyāna)* goes beyond effortlessness. The distinction between the subject, object and their relationship disappears. There is no feeling or awareness of being apart from anything. One does not practice *samādhi.* Effort or practice is involved only up until meditation. The doer disappears in *samādhi.* One simply is in *samādhi*, i.e. cognitive absorption. Initially this may involve a breathless state of communion with the Lord. After experiencing this frequently it may begin to permeate our mind during waking and sleeping states.

Practice: Start with the *haṁsa* meditation, gradually allowing the space between the breaths and the space between the thoughts to grow. Later learn and practice the *samādhi kriyās* as taught in the *Babaji's Kriya Yoga* level III initiation.

4. *trayam-ekatra saṃyamaḥ*

traya = of the three

ekatra = upon one object, in one place, in close connection; together, taken all together

saṃyama = literally: thorough restraint; from *sam*: thorough, great, com, con; and *yama:* restraint: (see verse II.29) here interpreted as "communion" or "constraint."

The practice of these three [*dhāraṇā, dhyāna and samādhi*] together upon one object is communion [*saṁyama*].

When concentration, meditation and samadhi are combined in a single practice, it may be termed "thorough restraint," "constraint" or "communion." Often translators have referred to *samyama* as "constraint." The Sanskrit suffix "*sam*" is similar in meaning to the English suffix "com" or "con," indicating "thoroughly" or "greatly." As will be seen in the following verses, *samyama* involves various elements, objects and ideas, bringing about mundane or superhuman attainments (*siddhis*). In this context, this relation with various objects may be best interpreted by the term "communion."

In such a state of communion (*saṁyama)* with the object of contemplation, Divine power flows towards whatever object or idea one focuses upon, and thus it manifests spontaneously. Just as in the microcosm of the human body one need only give the suggestion to raise the arm for it to rise, in the macrocosm made accessible by *saṁyama* the Divine powers manifest at will.

Practice: Do everything with firm intention, visualizing clearly what is to be done. Do everything calmly, allowing the universe to work its will through you.

5. *taj-jayāt prajñā-ālokaḥ*

tad = that; this

jayāt = because of, due to the mastery; conquering, triumph *prajñā* = discernment; understanding; insight (see I.20)

āloka = light, lustre, splendour; looking, seeing, beholding

Due to the mastery [of communion] the light of insight arises.

In verse I.20 insight (*prajñā*) is one of five developments preceding the realization of undistinguished cognitive absorption (*asamprajñāta-samādhi*). It is not ordinary knowledge, based on mental experience or intellectual reasoning, but an illumined type, born of inspiration and coming down from the psychic or transcendent spheres of human consciousness. It is knowing something because one "is" that something. These were discussed in the commentary on verse I.42 and I.44.

Practice: Ask the Lord "What do you want me to do?" Practice the *Babaji saṁyama dhyāna-kriyā* regularly whenever you need guidance.

6. *tasya bhūmiṣu viniyogaḥ*

tasya = its

bhūmiṣu = in or at stages; established; grounded; earth

viniyoga = application, progression

Its progression is in stages.

Cognitive insights come gradually and may be associated with material or abstract supports as indicated in verses I.42 and I.44. As mentioned in verse I.17 object-oriented cognitive absorption (*saṁprajñātaḥ samādhiḥ)*, may be accompanied by observations, reflections, rejoicing and the experience of "I am." With renewal it gradually becomes stabilized and purified.

Practice: Regularly practice all of the *dhyāna kriyās* taught in *Babaji's Kriya Yoga* level I initiation. Record the insights you receive in a journal.

7. *trayam-antar-aṅgaṃ pūrvebhyaḥ*

traya = three; tripartite; three part

antar = internal

aṅga = limb

pūrvebhyāḥ = [compared to the] preceding [*yogas*]

[Compared to the] preceding limbs, [these] three [together] are the inner limbs [of].

This verse refers to the eight limbs, or members, of *aṣṭāṅga Yoga* cited in verse I.29. The first limbs, namely, restraint (*yama)*, observation (*niyama)*, posture (*āsana*), breath control (*prāṇāyāma)* and sense withdrawal (*pratyāhāra*) govern the *yogin's* external relationships, through the physical body and in relationship with the external world. The last three members; concentration (*dhāraṇā)*, meditation (*dhyāna*) and cognitive absorption (*samādhi)* deal with consciousness itself, and so are deemed to be more internal.

As we work more internally we begin to let go of our need to be separate and "special." These practices begin to free us from being self-centered and acting out of egoistic motivations. With these practices of meditation and contemplation we become more aware of a universal inclusiveness. When we begin to experience union with something far greater than ourselves we begin to have the desire to be released from impulses, instincts and the mind's petty movements.

Practice: Regularly practice discrimination. Notice in every action any motivation or feeling which comes from the ego.

8. *tad-api bahir-aṅgaṃ nirbījasya*

tad = that

api = also, even, indeed

bahir = outer, external

aṅgaṁ =limbs

nirbījasya =of the seedless

These three are indeed the outer limbs of the seedless cognitive absorption [*samādhi*].

However, in relation to seedless cognitive absorption (*nirbīja samādhi,* see verse I.51) these last three limbs or members are external, mere aids to be eventually surpassed.

Thus said Sri Aurobindo: "When the inner Self which is the source of the spiritual aspiration comes to the forefront, and it pulls consciousness into itself, peace, ecstasy, freedom, wideness, the opening to light and higher knowledge begins to naturally, spontaneously emerge."

<u>Practice</u>: Develop purity in feelings whether it is in sympathy, in love, etc. Experience true feeling without ulterior motivation. Notice every feeling, which comes up; be aware of any ego-based motivation, which may lie beneath it.

9. *vyutthāna-nirodha-saṃskārayor abhibhava-prādurbhāvau nirodha-kṣaṇa-citta-anvayo nirodha-pariṇāmaḥ*

vyutthāna = arising, the action of being turned outward, restless

nirodha = cessation (see I.2); subsiding

saṃskārayoḥ = of the residual impressions; impression left by past action which conditions future actions; impressions which reside in the subconscious

abhibhava = overpowering, powerful

prādurbhavau = appearance, manifestation,

nirodha = cessation, restraint

kṣaṇa = moment, instant

citta = consciousness; mind

anvayoḥ = following, succession, connection

nirodha = cessation, restraint

pariṇāmaḥ = transformation; engagement; development

When the restless [movements] arising within consciousness are overpowered and subside [by the action] of restraint, there follows, in that moment, the development of the subconscious impression of restraint.

Verses III.9 to III.15 deal with the nature of change or transformation. Unlike some of the later classical texts like the *Upaṇiṣads,* which considers all change to be unreal, both Patañjali and the *Tirumantiram* consider change to be real. Consciousness (*citta)* is the constant, but its contents are continually changing. So also Nature (*prakṛti*) is the constant, in which various manifestations come and go. Here, *nirodha,* or cessation, refers to ceasing the false identification with what is transient, that is egoism. The process of cleansing egoism was described in the commentaries of verse I.2 and I.12.

Sri Aurobindo speaks of this as the "purifying movement of Shiva."**(1)** At a certain stage without any apparent reason, one loses his or her interest in the world and life in it. But that indifference, when established on a purer level of consciousness, becomes the bliss of oneness, love and sympathy and fellowship. There is a change, where the old form of these movements drops off, leaving room for a new higher Self to express itself. During transition and change, there is a vacuum created, which expresses itself as disappointment. But expansion can fill it. This new nature creates a stable foundation for lasting Bhakti and Bliss.

Practice: 1. *śuddhi dhyāna kriyā,* as taught in *Babaji's Kriya Yoga* level I.; 2. When the heart opens, turn toward the Divine alone, and keep its essential purity. When opening to higher consciousness be still, and avoid being dispersed in mental movements. Do not want for anything, not even understanding of what is happening.

10. *tasya praśānta-vāhitā saṁskārāt*

tasya = its

praśānta = calm

vāhitā = flow

saṁskārāt = habit

The calm flow of cleansing transformation develops through subconscious impressions.

By cultivating the practice of detachment (see verses I.2 and I.12) a subconscious habit pattern *(saṁskāra)* of detachment *(vairāgya)* gradually forms. In this way one automatically "lets go" of the egoistic tendency to identify with objects of attention, thoughts and emotions. As indicated in I.17, when this non-attachment is complete, there is no more effort made to detach. One is detached and without desire. Supreme peace reigns.

When we begin to be aware of another consciousness other than the ego and truly begin to live within its influence more and more, then the purifying actions happen on a continuous and self-sustaining basis.

Practice: When experiencing peace, joy or love, realize what it is, and trace it to its Source. Repeat the experience over and over until it is settled in your being.

11. *sarva-arthatā-ekāgratayoḥ kṣaya-udayau cittasya samādhi-pariṇāmaḥ*

sarva = all

arthatā = meaning, object; thingness, objectivity

ekāgratayoḥ = one-pointedness

kṣaya = declining; destruction

udayau = arisen

cittasya = of mind, consciousness

samādhi-pariṇāmaḥ = development, engagement or modification in samadhi

When there is a decline in objectification and [there is an] appearance of one-pointedness, [there arises] the development of the cognitive absorption [*samādhi*] of the mind.

The mind in its ordinary state is outwardly distracted by "all objects" through the five senses and their subtle counterparts (through imagination). The *yogin* cultivates concentration (*dhāraṇā)* and one-pointedness (*ekāgrataḥ*) and turns the consciousness inward, until it becomes absorbed in one single object, be it a subtle one or the Self.

Practice: Practice the second *dhyāna kriyā (eka rūpa* or "one-form" as taught in the *Babaji's Kriya Yoga* level I initiation. When working, concentrate on one task at a time. In daily life, remain centered, inwardly focused as a witness.

12. *tataḥ punaḥ śānta-uditau tulya-pratyayau cittasya-ekāgratā-pariṇāmaḥ*

tataḥ = then, from that; hence

punaḥ = again, repeated

śānta = subdued, quieted, appeased, pacified, calm, undisturbed

udita = arisen, apparent, visible

tulya = equal, same, equal, of the same kind, similar

pratyaya = thoughts that direct awareness; intention

cittasya = of consciousness

ekāgratā = one-pointedness

pariṇāma = transformation; modification; development

Hence, when the intentions that direct the repeated arising and subsiding [of thoughts] become similar, there is a transformation [into a] one-pointedness of consciousness.

Here Patañjali elaborates on the process of transformation (*pariṇāma)* from ordinary dispersed consciousness to cognitive absorption *(samādhi).*

"Why should that steady-minded one who knows the object of perception to be in its very nature nothing, consider one thing acceptable and another unacceptable?" (*Aṣṭavakra Saṁhitā* III.13). The only thing that really affects us is what we think about things. Who do our thoughts really affect? When we identify with the body, the senses, the eyes that see and the ears that hear; what are we really experiencing? Even when we think only of the Divine, sometimes our eagerness produces restlessness in the mind, which blocks our progress.

Practice: Cultivate equanimity in the face of duality, gain or loss, success or failure, praise or blame, pleasure or pain.

13. *etena bhūta-indriyeṣu dharma-lakṣaṇa-avasthā-pariṇāmā vyākhyātāḥ*

etena = by or with this

bhūta = elements: earth, water, fire, air, space; constituent of the manifest world

indriya = sense organ; power

dharma = essential character

lakṣaṇa = characteristic; time factor

avasthā = stability, stage, condition

pariṇāma = transformation; engagement; evolution, ripeness, result *vyākhyātāḥ* = explained, fully detailed

By this, concerning the sense organs and the elements, the transformation of the quality, character and condition [of the mind] have been fully detailed.

Patañjali describes how changes occur in three ways: (1) change in its substance or qualities (*dharma-pariṇāma*); (2) chronological, i.e. past, present and future (*lakṣana-pariṇāma*); (3) overall condition with stages of growth or decay (*avasthā-pariṇāma*). For example, the substance clay may in the present be in the form of a water jar; in the past it was simply a lump of clay; in future it will become dust at some point. These types of change are universal and occur in both material nature and with regards to the contents of consciousness. Just as clay is the constant in the above example, so consciousness is constant throughout the emerging of and detachment of thoughts.

During transformation (*pariṇāmaḥ)* there is much grinding and grating going on. There is a divine friction, which causes change to occur. We are not simply molded and shaped with loving hands; sometimes a chisel or hammer is necessary. Great determination and aspiration is needed. It is at those moments when we are being hammered that real progress can be made. But we must have a firm and determined will for realization.

Practice: Establish a regular discipline and keep at it. Cultivate awareness throughout all events.

14. *śānta-udita-avyapadeśya-dharma-anupātī dharmī*

śānta = quieted, calmed, undisturbed

udita = risen, ascended, born, produced,

avyapadeśya = not to be determined or defined

dharma = nature, character, essential quality

anupātī = following, corresponds to

dharmī = holder of the dharma; knowing or obeying the law, something subject to a particular state of condition

It is [that which is] subject to the particular laws of nature [i.e. *prakṛti*] [whose] nature is undisturbed, manifested, and undetermined.

A substance is present constantly, though different from its form or manifestation. The undisturbed forms are those that the substance has previously assumed. The manifested are those it now has, and the undetermined are those, which it will manifest in future. For example, the clay pot actually on the shelf was previously just a lump of earth. In future, after it breaks, it will undoubtedly be broken down into dust. Tirumūlar analyzes nature using as many as ninety-six elements (*tattvas*) (TM verse 154) as a means to ultimately transcending them. In TM verse 125 Tirumūlar states:

> *Siddhas* they that Śiva's world here visioned,
> *Nada* (sound principle) and *Nadanta* (ultimate sound)
> The Eternal, the Pure, reposing in Bliss unalloyed
> Thirty and six the steps to Liberation leading.

The "thirty and six" consists of five Śiva principles (*tattvas*), which arise in the pure immaterial sphere; seven principles of knowledge (*vidyā tattvas)* arising in the immaterial/material sphere, and twenty-four (*prakṛti tattvas)* arising in pure material sphere. Underlying this analysis is the assumption that by understanding the nature of what binds one's consciousness, one may liberate one's Self from it ultimately.

Practice: Practice the *īnai (Tam.) rūpa,* literally "moving form"), Fourth, (*arūpa* or formless), Fifth (*pūrṇa bhāva,* literally "emotion-filled"*)* and Advanced *dhyāna kriyās,* taking as the object each of the thirty-six *tattvas.*

15. *krama-anyatvaṁ pariṇāma-anyatve hetuḥ*

krama = sequences, series, succession, order

anyatvam = differentiation; otherness

pariṇāma = development, transformation; evolution

anyatve = in the or concerning the otherness or difference

hetu = cause; reason

The differentiation in the sequences [of these different phases] is the cause of differences in [stages of] evolution.

Simply put, the myriad differences in the manifest world are caused by these three time based phases, as described in the previous verse. The universe cycles continuously. The nature of everything is that it exists, changes and is destroyed. The Self is not affected. Things get destroyed simply because of their own rigidity, but even then it isn't really destroyed. The essential elements remain the same in decay as in life. Things appear to go through disintegration in order to change form. The Universe arises from the Self, and dissolves back into the Self.

<u>Practice</u>: Consider that "everything that has ever existed and everything that will exist, is existing right now." And that: "Everything has one and the same constituent element; and everything lies in the interrelations." (The Mother)**(2)**

16. *pariṇāma-traya-saṃyamād-atīta-anāgata-jñānam*

pariṇāma = (stage of) evolution; transformation, ripeness, result

traya = three

saṃyamād = because of or due to communion

atīta = past

anāgata = future

jñānam = knowledge

From communion with the three-fold [stage of] evolution [arises] knowledge of the past and future.

Starting with this verse Patañjali describes how by practicing communion (*saṁyama*) on various objects or ideas, various powers are acquired, leading ultimately to the supreme realization of non-distinguished cognitive absorption (*asaṁprajñātaḥ samādhi*). In this verse he is referring to the three-fold nature of transformation or change *(pariṇāma)* discussed in verse III.13: external form, time variation and overall condition. In this case, for example a *yogin* adept at communion (*saṁyama*) could know the past, present and future of any person whom he chose to focus upon.

Let us look at all the powers of inner knowing in a pragmatic and practical way. The fact that some advanced *yogins* are able to read a person's past, present and future demonstrates Oneness: the oneness of matter. It is not so much that we should all aspire to have the power to know the future. If it pleases Him, we should know it, if not, what does it matter?

Practice: Allow yourself to feel connected to others, including friends, family and strangers alike. Love yourself and others. Be entirely nonjudgmental.

17. *śabda-artha-pratyayānām itara-itara adhyāsāt-saṁkaras tat-pravibhāga-saṃyamāt-sarva-bhūta-rūta-jñānam*

śabda = sound; word

artha = meaning; purpose

pratyayānām = of ideas

itara-itara = respective, reciprocal, one with another

adhyāsāt = because of superimposition

saṃkaraḥ = mixed together, confusion, co-mingling

tad = that

pravibhāga = distinction; separation, division

saṃyamāt = because of or due to communion

sarva = all

bhūta = being

rūta = sound, utterance, cry, noise, roar, yell, sound; resonance

jñānam = knowledge

Because of the superimposition of words, purposes and intentions with one another, [there arises] confusion; [however], through communion [focused on distinguishing them], knowledge of all things [is attained].

Generally, people do not make any distinction between an object, its word (*śabda*) name and sound (*rūta)* of the word. By communion (*saṁyama)* on this distinction, it is claimed the *yogin* can have knowledge of foreign languages. We should be aware of the powerful effect that words can have upon us. The effect corresponds to the meaning and to the intrinsic energy of the word. When the voice forms words, they can affect others. What we say and the words, which describe what we believe, can affect our reality.

Practice: Be conscious of the words you tell yourself and say to others. Imagine that they are powerful enough to create and establish themselves.

18. *saṃskāra-sākṣāt-karaṇāt-pūrva-jāti-jñānam*

saṃskāra = subconscious impressions

sākṣāt-karaṇāt = intuitive perception; actual feeling, immediate cause of anything

pūrva = previous

jāti = birth

jñānam = knowledge

Knowledge of previous births [arises] because of the intuitive perception of subconscious impressions.

In a state of communion (*saṁyama*), the adept may directly witness subconscious impressions and as a result see where they were formed, as a witness to the past. Thus even knowledge of previous births (*jāti)* becomes accessible.

It is generally not very useful to seek out previous birth information, as it may overwhelm one, due to the many painful experiences. However, if it comes spontaneously, it may provide useful insights. When one is firmly established in detachment (*vairāgya),* one can look more easily at previous birth information.

Practice: Practice the Memory Chain *dhyāna kriyā* as taught in the *Babaji's Kriya Yoga* level III initiation.

19. *pratyayasya para-citta-jñānam*

pratyayasya = of the intention

para-citta-jñānam = knowing the thoughts of another

[Similarly, because of the intuitive perception of another's] intention [one is capable of] knowing the thoughts of another.

The adept is able to read another person's mind, by practicing *saṁyama,* and tracing the perception of another's thought back to its source. While most ordinary persons may occasionally pick up the thoughts of others they generally ignore them, or confuse them with their own. However, the *yogin* sees that such thought forms come from outside himself, and by *saṁyama* is able not only to trace them back to their originator, but once inside, so to speak, read the present contents of another's mind. Until we have purified our own subconscious, however, it is not advisable to focus upon others or to attempt to read their thoughts, as this may simply strengthen our own negative tendencies, such as greed, lust, need for power or to manipulate. Even where one uses it to help or to heal, the *yogin* must respect the need for each person to work out his or her own *karma*. The *yogin*'s intervention may simply postpone the working out of another's karma. In general, the *yogin* does not intervene unless invited. Furthermore, most of the thoughts that people are having are not worth intercepting. So the *yogin* generally makes no effort to capture them.

Practice: Focus only upon the minds of great saints until your subconscious is purified.

20. *na ca tat-sa-ālambanaṃ tasya-aviṣayī-bhūtatvāt*

na = not

ca = and

tad = that, this

sālambanam = with a support or base; here: motive

tasya = its

aviṣayī = not having an object

bhūtatvāt = due to the state of being an element

But [knowing another's thoughts] is without [an actual] basis because there is no object in the elements.

In other words, the knowledge residing at the subtle level has no corresponding form in the manifest realm of the elements. There are limits to this mind reading. Patañjali here states that it does not extend to being able to see the external objects (*viṣaya)* which another may be experiencing or deriving his thoughts from.

Practice: See the Divine in everyone, that part of them which is universal, infinite and eternal.

21. *kāya-rūpa-saṃyamāt-tad-grāhya-śakti-stambhe cakṣuḥ-prakāśa-asaṃyoge' ntardhānam*

kāya = body

rūpa = form, one of the *tanmātras*

saṁyamāt = because of or due to the communion

tad = that

grāhya = to be grasped

śakti = power, here: capacity

stambhe = suspension, suppression, stoppage

cakṣus = eye

prakāśa = light

asaṃyoge = disruption; disjunction disunion

a*ntardhānam* = invisibility, hidden, concealed, invisible

Through communion on the form of the body, upon suspension of the capacity to be perceived, upon the disruption of light [traveling from that body] invisibility to the eye [follows].

Patañjali herein explains that if a *yogin* practices *saṁyama* on his own form and in so doing suspends the flow of light radiating from it, so that such light does not reach the eyes of others, he will in effect be invisible, or at least not noticed by others. Stories abound of how Saint Ramalinga in the latter part of the 19th century, after posing with a group of disciples before the photographer, left no impression on the photographic plates. A blank spot would invariably appear where he had been standing in the group. He himself stated that this was due to a Divine transformation of his body, rather than to any willful act of his own to be invisible.

Be humble, simple and introspective while working with conscientiousness and without attachment for reward or attention. Focus on the Oneness of all. Feel how intimately close we all are. These are ways to become invisible which might have some lasting value.

Practice: Practice humility, simplicity, and conscientious attention to your work.

22. *sa-upakramaṃ nir-upakramaṃ ca karma tat-saṃyamād-apara-anta-jñānam-ariṣṭebhyaḥ vā*

sa-upakramam = set in motion; undertaking; manifest

nir-upakramam = not in motion, not taken up, not pursued; latent

ca = and

karman = action

tat = that

saṃyamāt = because of or due to communion

apara-anta = time of death; latter end; conclusion; literally, "the Western extremity"

jñānam = knowledge

ariṣṭebhyaḥ = ill omens, signs of approaching death

vā = or

***Karma* is either latent or manifest. From communion on this or on the signs of approaching death, [arises] the knowledge of death.**

In verses II.12-14, the reservoir of *karmas*, types of *karmas*, and causes of *karma* were discussed. Here, by concentration on the reservoir of *karmas* lying deep in the subconscious, practicing *saṁyama*, the adept can see the trends and patterns, which will reveal his future, including the circumstances surrounding his or her death. Omens are external fortuitous or inopportune events which may signal events to come. While some may regard them as superstition, there is a science and art for reading them.

At times great *yogins* have foreseen death or other calamities, and through great effort have re-shaped the future. Great power is available to one who is at One with the Absolute. Even we as a collective consciousness can help to re-shape the future.

Practice: Do your sadhana not only for your own benefit, but also for the benefit of everyone, keeping in mind the words of the pledge in *Babaji's Kriya Yoga.*

23. *maitry-ādiṣu balāni*

maitry-ādiṣu = friendliness and so forth

balāṇi = powers; strengths

[By communion] on friendliness and other such qualities, the power [to transmit them is attained].

This verse refers to the attitudes recommended in verse I.33 including friendliness (*mettā*) towards the happy (*sukha*), compassion (*karuṇā*) towards the unhappy (*duḥkha*), delight (*muditā*) in the virtuous (*puṇya*), and equanimity (*upekṣā*) towards the non-virtuous (*apuṇya*). Such attitudes create calm in the mind, and set the stage for the development of power (*bala*). To ignore these attitudes would on the contrary incite, as it does in ordinary human consciousness, all sorts of dissipation of one's power through conflicts and unnecessary vital interchange and loss. Ordinary people fritter away their vital energy through thousands of unnecessary or unwise social activities or self defeating mental attitudes such as competition, jealousy, fear, anger, depression and pride, etc.

Practice: Be centered in gentleness and friendliness and manifest those qualities out to everyone you come into contact with. Genuinely smile at people as often as you can.

24. *baleṣu hasti-bala-ādīni*

bala = the strengh

hasti = elephant

bala = strengths; powers

ādini = others

[By communion] on the powers of elephants and other [such animals], their strength [is obtained].

By communion (*saṁyama*) on animals or phenomena in nature, like fire, wind, air, one acquires their characteristic power. For example, to acquire physical strength the elephant could be one's subject of meditation. In shamanistic traditions, such as in the American southwest, adepts will commune with native animals and manifest their special powers. This reflects the well-known principle of sympathetic vibrations in physics. We tend to become like what we think about. Those cultures with clearly formed ideals, or heroes, tend to replicate such heroes and heroic behavior. In contrast, in today's worldwide popular culture, our icons tend to be here today, gone tomorrow movie stars or sport celebrities. The result is a culture of cynicism, weakness and depression wherein lives are an extension of television and movies. To put it simply, "you are what you watch."

<u>Practice</u>: Contemplate the qualities of various animals that you feel attracted to. Allow yourself to absorb these qualities, cultivating affirmations, which invoke them.

25. *pravṛtty-āloka-nyāsāt sūkṣma-vyavahita-viprakṛṣṭa-jñānam*

pravṛtti = activity; moving onwards, advance, progress, coming forth, appearance, manifestation, cognition (see I.35); here: inner senses

āloka = light

nyāsāt = due to placing, setting, applying or casting

sūkṣma = subtle

vyavahita = concealed; obstructed

viprakṛṣṭa = remote; distant

jñānam = knowledge

By communion with the illuminated inner senses, the knowledge of the subtle, concealed and remote is obtained.

With reference to I.35, the term *pravṛtti* (cognition) and III.5 *āloka* (light), *pravṛtti-āloka* can be understood as "illuminated senses." They are generally not under our control and are not developed, except in the case of exceptional persons like clairvoyants. They are experienced by most persons during dreams, however. By communion (*saṁyoga)* on one or all of the inner senses, hidden knowledge related to what is subtle (*sūkṣma)* as atoms, hidden (*vyavahita)* as treasure, and remote (*viprakṛṣṭa)* as distant lands may be gained. Meditation generally requires some effort until inspiration brings experiences spontaneously.

Practice: Seek inspiration and illumination of the inner senses through regular practice of the *īnai rūpa dhyana kriya,* (literally "moving form") and *pūrṇa bhāva dhyana kriya,* (literally "emotion-filled"*)*, as taught in the *Babaji's Kriya Yoga* level I initiation.

26. *bhuvana-jñānaṃ sūrye saṃyamāt*

bhuvana = universe; world, cosmic region

jñānam = knowledge

sūrye = on the sun

saṃyamāt = because of, due to or owing to communion

From communion on the sun, knowledge of the world and cosmic regions is obtained.

This verse indicates how the adepts were able to explore the universe, as evidenced in their works on astronomy and astrology. It is helpful to acquire our astrological natal chart. The Vedic system of recording indicates what your soul has promised to do in this lifetime, and lessons to be learned. Some commentators, such as Swami Hariharananda Aranya have argued that the word "sun" here refers to the "solar entrance" in the human body, and he has explained that this is the central energy channel (*suṣumna nāḍī),* which lies in the spinal column, and extends to the crown.(3) As the human body is a microcosmic replica of the macrocosm, when practicing *saṁyama* on this ray of effulgent light, the whole universe is revealed. He goes onto explain the seven regions of the world, as first described by the Sage Vyāsa: (1) the region of the truth (*satya-loka*); (2) the region of austerity (*tapas-loka*); (3) the people's region (*jana-loka*); (4) the region of the great Prajāpati, Brahma, the Creator (*mahar-loka*); (5) region of the great god Indra (*mahar-indra-loka*); (6) an intermediate region extending to the pole star (*antarikṣa-loka*); and (7) the ethereal region attached to this earth region, where the souls of humans go after death (*bhu-loka*).

With the elimination of the fluctuations of the mind (*cittavṛttiḥ),* one may realize the existence of different heavenly regions (*lokas).* At the time of death, if one leaves by way of the "solar entrance," the *suṣumna,* one attains to the higher astral regions of the *devas* or beyond in the causal regions of truth. This is known as great cognitive absorption (*mahā-samādhi*), wherein the *yogin* exits through the crown. Otherwise one exits through the "lunar entrance," that is, one of the nine openings of the body (genital, anus, two eyes, two ears, two nostrils, mouth), depending upon the responses to desires existing at the end of one's life. If one exits through the subtle anus or genital openings, for example, one may suffer in the lower astral planes. There, while the mind is active and full of desires, these cannot be realized because without sense organs one has no power to act.

27. *candre tārā-vyūha-jñānam*

candre = on the moon

tārā = stars

vyūha = ordering, arrangement, distribution

jñānam = knowledge

[By communion] on the moon [comes] knowledge [of the] stars' arrangements.

Similarly, by communion (*saṁyama)* with the moon, adepts were able to gain knowledge of not only its influences on us but that of distant stars and constellations. The *Siddhas* developed the science of *Svara Yoga,* which includes using the influence of the moon on our subtle and physical bodies. It affects right and left nostril breathing, the right and left hemispheres of the brain, women's menstrual and fertility cycles, not to mention the movement of the tides and electromagnetic and psychic influences.

Swami Haraharananda Aranya has identified the "moon" here as referring to the "lunar opening," the senses, and has emphasized that those who do not exit their body by the *suṣumna* or "solar opening," as discussed in the previous verse, must reincarnate on earth.**(4)**

Practice: Notice the periods where lunar breathing and creative, spatial, visual thinking and imagination are predominant.

28. *dhruve tad-gati-jñānam*

dhruve = on the the polar star

tad = that [refers to stars in the previous *sūtra*]

gati = movement; motion

jñānam = knowledge

[By communion] on the pole star comes knowledge [of the] stars' movements.

Similarly, by communion (*saṁyama)* with the polestar, knowledge of the stars' movements is gained. As it maintains its position in the sky, it serves as a reference point. By fixing one's attention on a single point like the polestar, while maintaining stillness and simultaneously becoming engrossed in the sky, the movement of the stars will be known.

29. *nābhi-cakre kāya-vyūha-jñānam*

nābhi = central point; navel

cakre = on the wheel

kāya = body

vyūha = arrangement

jñānam = knowledge

[By communion] on the wheel of the navel, knowledge of the body's constitution is obtained.

By practicing communion (*saṁyama*) on the solar plexus or navel chakra, (*nābhi-cakra)* the subtle anatomy of the human body can be traced. This *cakra* is the center of the power of action. The *yogin* adepts identified as many as 72,000 channels (*nāḍīs*) radiating through the human body in its physical and subtle dimensions. Several important *nāḍīs* are the object of specific practices in *Yoga.*

The Mother suggests that through study of the navel center we might discover our purpose, or sense of life. She suggests that the way to connect to this area is to draw the vital breath (*prāṇa)* around the umbilical region and relax. Draw "a quiet ease" in with this vital breath. Imagine this *prāṇa* widening the cramped area. Relax and let go. "Imagine catching hold of a wave movement and relax. Float on that infinite undulating movement."**(5)**

Practice: Practice the above technique of widening around the navel center. Do not complain about the work life has given you to do. Cultivate an optimistic attitude. See your life and work in a new light.

30. *kaṇṭha-kūpe kṣut-pipāsā-nivṛttiḥ*

kaṇṭha = throat

kūpe = well; hollow, cavity

kṣudh = hunger

pipāsā = thirst

nivṛttiḥ = cessation, disappearance

[By communion] on the throat cavity, cessation of hunger and thirst is achieved.

The *viśuddhi cakra*, located in the throat, is the center of visualization. Hunger and thirst is primarily a function of one's imagination and habit. Eating and drinking provides immediate gratification and gives relief to emotional suffering, such as depression or frustration. However, by pacifying this emotional need through neutralization of the throat *cakra (viśuddhi cakra)* directly, the impulse to eat and drink may be largely eliminated.

Practice: *mantras, āsanas, dhyāna kriyās* designed to awaken the throat *cakra*. Let go of desire. Control emotional promptings to eat or drink. Eat only when you are hungry. Communicate your feelings.

31. *kūrma-nāḍyāṃ sthairyam*

kūrma = tortoise

nāḍī = subtle energy channel; pathway of *prāṇa* in the body

sthairyam = motionlessness; firmness; stability

[By communion] on the tortoise channel, motionlessness [is achieved].

The tortoise channel (*kūrma nāḍī*) is one of the major energy channels (*nāḍīs*) in the vital body. It is situated below the throat. *Saṁyama* on it brings about motionlessness or steadfastness during meditation.

The tortoise symbolizes the place where heaven and earth meet. The upper shell of the tortoise is the symbol for heaven and its square underside is the symbol for earth. It is associated with the lunar cycle, the primal mother, and the primal essence. As we begin to see the connectedness of things, we realize that the way to heaven is through earth.

Practice: Put the epicenter of the mind on this tortoise channel (*kūrma nāḍī*), using the Sixth *dhyāna kriyā* (*nāḍī dhyāna*) and experience inner stillness.

32. *mūrdha-jyotiṣi siddha-darśanam*

mūrdha = the head

jyotiṣi = on the light; brightness

siddha = perfected one, accomplished one

darśanam = vision

[By communion] on the light [at the crown of] the head, a vision of perfected ones is obtained.

Each person has a radiance around the physical body. When it develops through the progressive practice of *Yoga*, an intense light may be seen around the head, particularly above the head. We are not limited to the physical body. Above the crown of the head lies the seat of the Supreme Being. By *saṁyama* on the light at the top of the head we may have visions of supreme masters and adepts and other divine beings. In *Tirumantiram* verse 194:

> The bee, that nectar seeks, flies high for its flower on top,
> And therefore, it sucks the fragrant juice;
> Even so, they who seek the blessed grace divine,
> Aspire for the Light beyond visible reach of our eyes.

When you penetrate the light (*jyotis*) above the crown of the head (*mūrdha*), there is no difference between the subject and object, except as your individuality is given expression with imagination. For the majority of students of *Yoga*, the light of the perfected ones is readily available, even without perfecting this technique. The light shines from the written words of the perfected ones. It is a tangible light you can plunge into every time you pick up their book to read. Sri Aurobindo says, "The Word has power - even the ordinary written word has power. If it is an inspired word it has still more power. What kind of power it has depends on the nature of the inspiration and the theme and the part of the being it touches. If it is the Word itself - as in certain utterances of the great Scriptures, Veda, Upanishads, Gita, it may well have a power to awaken a spiritual and uplifting impulse, even certain kinds of realization."

Practice: Devotedly study the sacred books of the Enlightened and Perfected Ones. There is a personal day-to-day guidance and inspiration there for you. Their guidance will come to you at the perfect moment. Practice *Svarupa Jyoti Samadhi Dhyana Kriya* as taught in Babaji's Kriya Yoga Third level initiation.

33. *prātibhād-vā-sarvam*

prātibhād = flash of illumination; intuition; spontaneous and unmediated flash of intuition

vā = or

sarvam = everything

Or, all [the powers come by themselves through] a flash of illumination.

The flash of illumination (*prātibha)* is an experience, a sample of what may come later: lasting enlightenment, or undistinguished cognitive absorption (*asaṁprajñātaḥ samādhi*). That is, even without practicing *saṁyama,* such powers may come spontaneously, as accompaniments to the flash of illumination. The obscurity of normal human consciousness is blown away in such an infusion of light and consciousness.

When Sri Aurobindo was asked if the method of sitting in vacant meditation to see what comes from the intuitive gods and goddesses was effective, he said "that is the way things are supposed to come. When the mind becomes quiet, an intuition, perfect or imperfect, is supposed to come hopping along and jump in and look around the place. Of course, it is not the only way. I wrote everything I have written since 1909 in that way, or rather through a silent mind, and not only a silent mind, but a silent consciousness. But gods and goddesses had nothing to do with it."**(6)**

Practice: Be aware of insight that comes to you when your mind is silent. One doesn't have to be seated in a perfect *āsana* to have a silent mind. We might be driving the car, or washing dishes, notice that mindless activity often opens us to receiving.

34. *hṛdaye citta-saṃvit*

hṛdaye = at the heart; the seat of feelings and sensations

citta = consciousness

saṃvid = knowledge; understanding

[By communion] at the heart, knowledge [of the nature of] consciousness [is obtained].

Consciousness (*citta)* manifests in the ordinary human being in only three states: physical (via the five senses), dream (whether in sleep or waking astral imagination), and dreamless sleep. There is a fourth (*turīya),* which is the fundamental transcendental state of awareness. This fourth state is accessible only by centering our attention at the heart; not the physical heart, but the center of our being, which, spatially exists in the middle of the chest. From that vantage point we may distinguish the other states of consciousness objectively; whereas usually one is simply absorbed by them, unaware.

Practice: Focus your concentration during meditation on the heart center (not the physical heart).

35. *sattva-puruṣayor-atyanta-asaṃkīrṇayoḥ pratyaya-aviśeṣaḥ bhogaḥ para-arthatvāt sva-artha saṁyamāt puruṣa-jñānaṃ*

sattva = beingness; product of *prakṛti;* here: manifest being in nature

puruṣa = the Self; inactive witness; soul; human, primeval human as source of everything

atyanta = perfect, endless, unbroken, perpetual, excessive, very great

asaṃkīrṇa = unmixed, not unclean, not confused; pure

pratyaya = awareness; intention; fundamental notion; fundamental notion

aviśeṣo = indistinct

bhogaḥ = experience; use, application, resultant experience

para = opposite, ulterior, farther than, more than, superior or inferior to

artha = object, aim, purpose, goal

para-arthatvāt = because of [being] dependent on someone else; the highest advantage; here: ulterior motive

sva-artha = own purpose; for its own sake

saṃyama = communion

puruṣa = Self; human, primeval human as source of everything

jñānam = knowledge

[When there is] an ulterior motive, the resultant experience is [that there is] no distinction [between] the awareness of manifest being in nature and the Self; [when one practices] communion for its own sake, [one obtains] Self-knowledge.

Nature (*prakṛti*) has three modes of manifestation (*tri-guṇas),* namely: activity *(rajas)*; inertia *(tamas)* and being (*sattva). Sattva* also implies balance, equanimity and includes the most subtle part of manifest nature: the intellect. In ordinary human consciousness, because of the veil of ignorance, there is a confusion or lack of distinction between our pure Self, which is uninvolved in the manifestation and our body-mind complex. By communion *(saṁyama)* on this distinction between the Pure Self (*puruṣa)* and the manifestation of Nature *(prakṛti)* at the subtlest level of our being (*sattva*), we may understand what is the Self.

Practice: While reading, studying and pondering with the intellect, allow the inner consciousness to remain aware and apart, witnessing the play of words and ideas. Learn and practice *nityānanda kriyā* as taught in *Babaji's Kriya Yoga* level II initiation.

36. *tataḥ prātibha-śrāvaṇa-vedanā-ādarśa-āsvāda-vārtāḥ jāyante*

tatas = thence

prātibha = intuition; divination; here: spontaneous flashes of intuition

śrāvaṇa = hearing, relating to or perceived by the ear

vedanā = touching , feeling, sensing

ādarśa = seeing, act of perceiving by the eyes

āsvāda = tasting, enjoying, eating

vārtā = smelling

jāyante = are born or are produced

Thus, spontaneous intuitive flashes [based in] hearing, touching, seeing, tasting, and smelling are produced.

With reference to verse III.35, the knowledge of the Self, gained by communion *(saṁyama)* on the distinction between the Self (*puruṣa)* versus Being (*sattva),* may produce the powers of clairvoyance, clairaudience, clairsentience, etc. When one is identified with the Self, which is Divine, then its power flows through the latent subtle faculties.

Practice: Cultivate inner vision and hearing using the *īnai rūpa,* (literally "moving form") *dhyana kriya* and *pūrṇa bhāva,* (literally "emotion-filled") *dhyana kriya,* as taught in the *Babaji's Kriya Yoga* level I initiation, as well as the advanced *kriyās* related to the *siddhis.*

37. *te samādhāu-upasargāḥ vyutthāne siddhayaḥ*

te = these [*siddhis*]

samādhau = in cognitive absorption

upasargāḥ = impediment, obstacle, trouble

vyutthāne = rising up, awakening, yielding, giving way; here: in the waking state

siddhayaḥ = attainments, success, performance, fulfillment, perfection

These attainments are obstacles to cognitive absorption but are accomplishments in the waking state.

One should not become attached to these accomplishments (*siddhis),* however marvelous they may be from the worldly perspective. Making them one's goal will only delay the perfection of cognitive absorption (*samādhi).* Let them come but let them go. They are mere signposts along the way, and are by no means necessary.

The Mother: on accomplishments (*siddhis*): "all those powers, gifts, constructions, manifestations, it all reminded me of the life of a traveling juggler. It's like a juggler's life - you go from fairground to fairground, displaying your feats of skill. There was a time when I saw all these things as something very nice, for widening my power of imagination so I could present these things to the Lord. But it is not necessary." There is excitement, it is like champagne bubbles, but it complicates things, it clouds the issue. You have to wait for the bubbles to subside before you can calmly set off again on your way toward the goal.

Practice: Practice *Yoga* without attachment to the results.

38. *bandha-kāraṇa-śaithilyāt pracāra-saṃvedanāt ca cittasya para-śarīra-āveśaḥ*

bandha = binding, holding, bondage

kāraṇa = cause, reason, motive, origin

śaithilyāt = because of or from relaxation

pracāra = coming forth, showing oneself, manifestation, appearance

saṃvedanāt = because of, from or due to the knowledge

ca = and

cittasya = of the mind or consciousness

paraśarīra = another body or embodiment

āveṣaḥ = entrance, taking possession of, entering

Due to the relaxation of the cause of bondage and the knowledge of manifestation, entering into another body of consciousness [can take place].

This is known as *prāpti* and is one of the eight great powers enumerated in several texts of *Yoga* including the *Tirumantiram* verse 668:

To become tiny as the atom within the atom (*animan)*
To become big in unshakeable proportions (*mahiman*)
To become light as vapor in levitation (*laghiman*)
To enter into other bodies in transmigration (*prāpti*)
To be in all things, omni-pervasive (*prākāmya*)
To be Lord of all creation in omnipotence (*īṣita)*
To be everywhere in omnipresence (*vaṣitā)*
To consummate any wish or desire (*kāmâvasāyitā*)
These eight are *siddhis* Great

In his "Oceanic Life Story" poem the *Siddha* Pōkanāthar (pronounced

Boganathar) describes how he transmigrated into another body to accomplish his mission in China. Tirumūlar himself relates how he transmigrated into the body of the dead cowherd Mūlan. (TM 68)

This was done to fulfill their duty (*dharma*). Boganathar was asked by his guru Kalaṇgi Nāthar to take over his mission in China, and after beginning his work there he realized the need to change his body in order to fulfill the work. Tirumūlar also speaks of the mission Śiva gave to him in the south of India, and how this required his transmigration into the body of the dead cowherd *Moolar.* While we probably will never be called to transmigrate into another body in this life, we may all prepare for our next birth by visualizing it, seeking inspiration, and arranging our present inventory of *karma* to facilitate it.

Practice: Allow the Divine's plan to fulfill Itself through you. Visualize the ideal conditions of your next incarnation.

39. *udāna-jayāt-jala-paṅka-kaṇṭaka-ādiṣu asaṅga utkrāntiś-ca*

udāna = the vital force in the upper part of the body; up breath, one of the five vital breaths; the emitting of the breath in an upward direction.

jayāt = because of, from or owing to mastery; victory

jala = water

paṅka = mud

kaṇṭaka = thorn

ādisu = and so forth

asaṅgaḥ = unattached, free from ties, independent; imperviousness

utkrāntiḥ = gone forth or out; gone over or beyond; here: levitation

ca = and

By mastery over the vital force in the upper part of the body [the adept gains the power of] imperviousness to water, mud and thorns [as well as the power of] levitation.

The flow of life force *(prāṇa),* is classified according to the five regions of the body: (1) the heart region (*prāṇa)*; (2) the abdominal region (*samāna)*; (3) pelvic region and legs (*apâna*); (4) head and neck (*udāna*); (5) *vyāna*: pervading all parts of the body. Communion (*saṁyama)* with the life force in the upper part of the body enables physical levitation, also known as laghima, and is one of the eight great *siddhis* cited in TM 668.

The Mother says, breath control (*prāṇāyāma)* with the idea of gaining powers fouls things up more than anything. Do *prāṇāyāma* simply as a help to your progress. Directing *prāṇa* into unwell areas of the body is very beneficial, and is known in *Babaji' s Kriya Yoga* level II initiation as *prāṇa sahitchay kriyā.* Mastery over the vital forces (the various kinds of *prāṇa),* the Mother says, is like the Lord entering into the body as air, and when it is held inside like that all the air begins to flow out into everybody and does its work in each one, with such a sensation of ease, of tranquil power, and assuredness; so comfortably peaceful.**(7)** While ascetics undoubtedly may become physically impervious to disturbance by thorns, mud, insects etc, symbolically, we might interpret the water, as the emotions, the mud, as that which covers the light of the Self, and the thorns, as the thorny path, which becomes painful when we make false steps, returning to old bad psychological habits.

Practice: 1. Practice *prāṇa satchitchay kriyā,* and the other *kriyās* related to self-healing, as taught in *Babaji' s Kriya Yoga* level II and III initiations. 2. Practice *śuddhi dhyāna kriyā* and sense withdrawal (*pratyāhāra)* during deep meditations, as in the level I initiations. 3. When you discover disturbances within you, say: "Lord, it is up to you to rid me of these habits. I cannot do it on my own." Once these things leave us we have a change in consciousness. At that point we should feel "lighter than air."

40. *samāna-jayāj-jvalanam*

samāna = vital force in the abdominal area of the body

jayāt = because of mastery

jvalanan = glow, radiance

By mastery of the vital force in the abdominal region [here is] radiance.

This may occur as a result of communion (*saṁyoga)* with the life force (*prāṇa*) in this region (*samāna)*, or as a result of breathing which activates the solar plexus. The reservoir or vital sheath, which surrounds the physical body, is filled. As one ages, normally this reservoir is depleted and the aura becomes progressively duller or even discolored when there is illness.

Compare this to TM verse 689:

> In the days the *Siddha* stands thus in Self control (*vaṣitvā)*
> Radiant as the Sun,
> If he attains the rare vision of the True Being
> Golden becomes His body
> Dead his sense organs,
> And he visions the śakti
> That like a tender vine appears.

By combining the *prāṇa*; which is upward flowing, and that within the pelvic region and legs (*apâna*),which is downward flowing, and moving both upwards, the fire of *tapas* begins to magnetize the body and the aura builds.

Practice: Practice *kriyā kuṇḍalinī prāṇāyāma* as a way of developing vibrant health, radiance, and strength.

41. *śrotra-ākāśayoḥ saṃbandha-saṃyamād-divyaṃ śrotram*

śrotra = ear

ākāśayoḥ = and ether

saṃbandha = relationship, connection, union

saṃyamāt = because of, due to, or owing to communion

divyam = divine

śrotram = hearing, here, *divyam-śrotam* is "clairaudience"

[By communion] on the relationship between the ear and ether, there is clairaudience.

Sound travels through the media of ether or space. In clairaudience, one separates the sense of hearing from the sense organ, the ear, and mentally shifts the center of consciousness to a distant place, "across space" so to speak. One then listens to the sounds that arise. It requires much practice, as a method, though it may come spontaneously (as in verse III.33).

It is useful to develop the natural capacities of our subtle senses. The method of developing the subtle sense of clairaudience begins with the intention to do so. The Mother explains how we can "hear behind a sound," by contacting the subtle reality which lies behind the sound. You concentrate, and then hear what is behind it. It requires patient practice for many months.

Practice: Affirm your intention to become clairaudient. Practice the advanced *kriyās* taught in *Babaji's Kriya Yoga* level III initiation to develop it.

42. *kāya-ākāśayoḥ saṃbandha-saṃyamāt laghu-tūla-samāpatteḥ ca ākāśa-gamanam*

kāya = body

ākāśa = space, ether; the substratum of the quality of sound; a hole; zero

saṃbandha = relationship

saṃyamāt = because of or due to communion

laghu = light

tūla = cotton fiber

samāpatteḥ = because of or due to union; here: cognitive absorption

ca = and

ākāśa = space, ether; the substratum of the quality of sound; a hole; zero

gamanan = movement, going from

[By communion] on the relationship between the body and space, and [by being in a state of] cognitive absorption [focused upon] light [objects, such as] cotton, [the power to travel across] space [is gained].

This is another reference to levitation the power of lightness (*laghima*), discussed in verse III.38. Generally, in ordinary consciousness, we ignore ether, even though it is the fundamental background upon which the body and indeed all manifestations take place. By uniting (*samāpattiḥ)* one's consciousness and being with the ether (*ākāśaḥ)* the body (*kāya)* itself transcends the law of gravity and can move at will.

The Mother mentions how while bedridden she used to practice traveling across the space of several rooms to see what was happening in a studio there. She would be very still, shut her eyes, and gradually send out her consciousness. She did the exercise regularly, day after day, at a set hour. She suggests that we start with imagination and then it becomes fact. After awhile we sense the vision physically moving.**(8)**

Practice: Practice the *samādhi kriyās* taught during the *Babaji's Kriya Yoga* level III initiation, and while in that state, focus on a light object, such as cotton, silk or a feather.

43. *bahir-akalpitā vṛttir mahā-videhā tataḥ prakāśa-āvaraṇa-kṣayaḥ*

bahir = outer, external; unessential; outer limbs

akalpitā = inconceivable

vṛttiḥ = fluctuations [arising within consciousness, i.e. *citta-vṛttiḥ*]

mahā = great

videhā = bodilessness, incorporeal, death (see I.19)

tataḥ = hence; from there on, then, consequently

prakāśa = light

āvaraṇa = veil

kṣayaḥ = destruction; dwindling, a house; termination; more figuratively, "shedding"

During this great out of the body experience, the fluctuations arising within consciousness are inconceivable, as they are perceived to be external to this body, and from this, comes the dwindling of the veil over the light of the Self.

Because of egoism, we allow our consciousness to become involved in a cloud of thoughts, which is so thick it usually veils our true Self, which has the quality of light (*prakāśa).* By communion (*saṁyama)* with ether (*ākāśa,* as in verse III.41 and III.42) one transcends this cloud and sees the Light of the Self, which is behind it.

In referring to her truly great out-of-the-body experience, the Mother explained: "throughout the experience this present individuality no longer existed, this body no longer existed, there were no limits. I was no longer here - what was here was The Person. When she left the body it didn't mean that she left physical consciousness. Her overall contact with the terrestrial world remained the same. She explains, as soon as you rise to a certain height, the appearance of the body quickly loses its reality. There external appearance is very illusory. Our particular form, which we see with our physical eyes, is very superficial. From the vital world onwards, it is completely different.**(8)**

Practice: Practice the *samādhi kriyās,* taught in the *Babaji's Kriya Yoga* level III initiation, while contemplating this verse.

44. *sthūla-svarūpa-sūkṣma-anvaya-arthavattva-saṃyamād-bhūta-jayaḥ*

sthūla = gross, coarse, solid, material

svarūpa = own form, essence

sūkṣma = subtle

anvaya = correlative; connection; being linked to

arthavattva = purposefulness; significance, importance,

saṃyamāt = because of or due to communion

bhūta = elements

jaya = mastery

By communion with the objects [of nature] at their coarse and subtle levels and on their essence, correlations and purpose, mastery over the five elements is gained.

Objects (*viṣayāḥ)* in nature exist at various levels. At the coarse level, they can be perceived by the sense organs (*indriyāni*); they also have a typical form, which they take; they also stand in relation to other objects and serve some purpose.

We might say the elements of nature being earth (*pṛthvī),* water (*ap),* fire (*tejas),* air (*vāyu)* and ether (*ākāśa)* are distinct and different in composition. According to science, matter is energy in action. The Enlightened Ones say that energy (*prakriti)* is the force of Consciousness in action. Even though its presence is veiled, the Divine exists in all things. Everything exists in the Divine. The Divine brings things into existence in every possible combination. We see things in specific forms. We think a thing cannot both be and not be at the same time. Matter can be seen in the ordinary way and at the same time be perceived in another way.

Sri Aurobindo says: "Matter itself, you will one day realize, is not material, it is not substance, but a form of consciousness, *guṇa,* the result of quality of being, perceived by sense knowledge."**(9)**

Practice: The first *samādhi kriyā* taught during *Babaji's Kriya Yoga* level III initiation, while in communion with objects in nature.

45. *tato' ṇima-ādi-prādurbhāvaḥ kāya-saṃpat-tad-dharma-anabhighātaś-ca*

tataḥ = from that, thence, consequently

aṇima-ādi = the power of becoming minute as an atom and so forth

prādurbhāva = appearance; that which is visible

kāya = body

saṃpad = perfection, success, accomplishment;

tad = that

dharma = nature, character, essential quality, that which is established or held, virtue, religion

anabhighātaḥ = non-obstruction; unassailability, invulnerability

ca = and

Then [comes] the manifestation of powers such as bodily perfection and invulnerability of its functions.

Patañjali first refers to one of the famous eight great siddhis, known as, the power "to become tiny as the atom within the atom" (*aṇima).* The *Siddhas* were first-rate scientists and were able to explore not only the solar system, but also Nature at the subatomic particle level. Many of their findings correspond to those of modern day physics. By "others" he is referring to the other eight great powers, which are listed in the commentary on verse III.35 and in other texts of *Yoga* (see *Tirumantiram* verses 668-93 for an extensive description of these).

The traditional interpretations of these powers vary among the different texts. *Mahima* may mean the power to expand one's consciousness to the largest form or expanse. *Laghima* may mean the power of levitation, or to render the body light at will, or mastery over the element of air. *Prāpti* is the power of transmigration into another body or to extend the subtle body or its members (including astral travel), or the power to obtain any desired objective anywhere. *Prākāmya* is the power to be in all things, omni-pervasive; the power to derive enjoyment from everything heard or seen; the power to exercise an irresistible will on the minds of others; or the power to obtain a youthful appearance for an unusual length of time. *Vaśitva* is the power to be lord over all creation, the power to control and create, the power of mind over illusion (*māyā). Īśitṛtva* is the power to be everywhere in omnipresence; the power of command and control, resulting from non-attachment to objects. *Kāmāvasayitva* is the power to fulfill any wish or desire including the supreme desire, Self-realization; perfection of the body and invulnerability of its functions.

In numerous verses *Tirumūlar* speaks of this:

> The Fire I saw in *Kuṇḍalinī* radiates *Kālas* four;
> The *Prāṇa* I kindled and coursed through Centers Seven
> Pervades the body entire,
> With divine life that suffuses the fleshy body ambrosia,
> I grow into a tender fawn. (TM 738)

> They who effect the mystic union
> With the azure-hued *Śakti* within
> Will shed greying and wrinkling
> And regain youth for all to see;
> This I say is true, by Naṇḍi the Great. (TM 734)

> The breath that rose twelve *mātras* long,
> If you control and absorb within,
> well may you live a thousand years on land and sea,
> The body perishes not;
> True this is;
> Upon Lord of Naṇḍi, I declare. (TM 722)

Verses like these appear throughout the literature of the Eighteen Tamil *Yoga Siddhas,* who are legendary figures in the Dravidian culture of southern India, and who are reported to be still living after many hundreds of years.**(10)**

Instead of focusing on *siddhis* one may focus on evolutionary developments. These wonders of the world as we know it, what saints and masters have manifested, are examples that show us the capacity we have within ourselves to develop. These are seeds, which will blossom at the right time and place and within the right persons.

Sri Aurobindo and the Mother: "The physical and the subtle physical seem to fuse - as if they permeated one another. The physical material substance no longer has that unreceptive sort of density, which resists penetration. One vibration can change the quality of another. The subtle physical seems to dose out its power and light and capacity of consciousness according to the amount of receptivity in the purely physical vibration. Done very, very, gradually over a long period of time, but almost continuous work and mostly or only when the body is still, when all activity stops and the body is concentrated or immobile...or perhaps only passive the penetration is perceptible. It is visible. The penetration actually changes the composition. It is not merely a degree of subtlety. It is a change in the internal composition. Ultimately it has effect on the atomic level. And that is how the practical possibility of transformation can be accounted for. On the surface it is very humble work. Nothing sensational. No illuminations filing you with joy and that is fine for people seeking spiritual joys, but it belongs to the past. This is very modest work. The new combinations of vibrations are difficult for the body. The body must be very quiet, well under control, very peaceful or it panics. All the powers, *siddhis,* all the realizations, all these things are the grand extravaganza, the great spiritual spectacle. But this isn't like that. It is very modest, very unobtrusive, very humble, nothing showy about it. It takes years and years of silent, quiet, and extremely careful work before there are any tangible results, before anything can be noticed. As for those who want to go quickly, if they try going quickly in this realm they will be thrown off balance. You can't go quickly. Stubbornness is essential. The body is stubborn; and that is what is needed."**(11)**

Practice: *Svarupa (Soruba, Tam.) jyoti Samādhi Kriyā* and the technique of continuous bliss (*nityānanda kriyā*) as taught in *Babaji's Kriya Yoga* level III initiation, integrating them constantly with the subtle physical levels, quietly, patiently and stubbornly.

46. *rūpa-lāvaṇya-bala-vajra-saṃhananatvāni kāya-saṃpat*

rūpa = beauty; handsome form

lāvaṇya = gracefulness

bala = strength

vajra = thunderbolt, mighty, adamantine, hence implying indestructibility

saṃhananatvāni = having the quality of solidity, robustness, firmness; stability, endurability

kāyasaṃpat = perfection of the body

Beauty, grace, strength and extraordinary endurability [constitute] perfection of the body.

Patañjali here defines what he means by perfection of the body (see verse III.45) also known as *kaya siddhi* in the literature of the Tamil Yoga Siddhars. Rather than disparaging the body or emphasizing its mortality, Patañjali glorifies it with qualities that can only be called divine (*divyam*): beautiful (*rūpa)*, graceful (*lāvaṇya*), and enduring (*vajra-saṃhananatva).*

Tirumūlar speaks of "the attainment of the [perfection of] the body" (*kāya[saṁpat] siddhi*) in verses 724-796.

If he body perishes, *prāṇa* departs,
Nor will the Light of Truth be reached
I learned the way of preserving my body
And so doing, my *prāṇa* too. (TM 724)

So preservation of the body is not an end in itself, but a means to buy time to complete the process of Self-realization.

Time was when I despised the body
But then I saw the God within
And the body, I realized, is the Lord's temple
And so I began preserving it
With care infinite. (TM 725)

This famous verse ennobles the human body and promotes the care of it as an act of worship to the Supreme Being. The body is a sacred trust and the dwelling of the Lord.

> They who thus attained radiance a hundred-fold
> will live a thousand years in body robust
> And they who saw a thousand years thus
> May well live a million, trillion years. (TM 758)

Here he speaks of our potential to live in the body indefinitely. If the Divine is eternal and we realize the Divine, we also share this eternity.

> None know where the Lord resides;
> To them who seek Him
> He resides eternal within
> When you see the Lord
> He and you one become. (TM 766)

This last verse also encapsulates the philosophy of the Tamil *Siddhas* (*Saiva Siddhanta): Jīva* becoming *Śiva,* in contrast to the followers of the *Advaita Vedāntins* who would say "I am Brahman." To contrast the two points of view analogously, the latter view everything as though they were submerged in the ocean, whereas the former see things from the perspective of the wave on the surface of the ocean. To the *Advaita Vedāntins,* the world is unreal; to the *Saiva Siddhantins* it is real, but its form is temporary.

Our physical bodies are built in such a way that they instinctively attract painful experiences. To perfect the body means, one is able to face whatever hindrance, difficulty or evil, is drawn to it, and continue with confidence. Thoughts can have consequences in the body. Be aware of your physical state. When there is no reaction to a thought or an emotion in your body, not even sorrow, then you know there is perfection in the body.

To quote from Chapple and Viraj: " Perfection of the body does not arise in regard to a standard of health but proceeds from a comprehension of the operation of the *tattvas* (see *Bhagavad Gita XIII 2-5).*"**(12)**

Practice: Take time to reflect upon physical wellness. Be aware of what is happening in your body, including emotional sources of disturbances. Use the *nadi dhyāna kriyā* to discover hidden sources of ailments or disturbances, as taught in *Babaji's Kriya Yoga* level I initiation. Practice the 18 postures recommended by Babaji in his Kriyā *haṭha yoga.*

47. *grahaṇa-svarūpa-asmitā-anvaya-arthavattva-saṃyamād-indriya-jayaḥ*

grahaṇa = grasping; power of perception

svarūpa = its own form; essential nature

asmitā = ego; I-am-ness

anvaya = correlation; connection; association

arthavattva = significance; importance

saṃyama = because of , due to or owing to communion

indriya = sense organ; power of the senses, bodily power; eye, ear, nose, tongue and skin

jaya = mastery; conquest, victory, triumph; thus, *indriya-jayaḥ* is "victory or restraint over the bodily power of the senses."

By communion with the [power of] perception and on one's essential nature, as well as ego, their correlation and purpose, one gains mastery over the sense organs.

Previously, the senses were discussed in terms of sense withdrawal (*pratyāhāra*), from sources of distraction (verses II.54 and II.55). Here Patañjali says that one may master the senses, not by withdrawing or suppressing them, but in exploiting their full potential. This may occur by fully understanding, through communion with the power of perception, the purpose of the senses, their relationship to our true Self, and to our ego. Generally, we ignore this relationship, as we are simply involved in whatever sensory input they give us. This verse is parallel in focus to III.44, but while the gross level of being is linked to the elements, in this *sutra*, the subtle sense of ego/I-am-ness is linked to the sense organs.

When we study our nature, we are able to see which subconscious impressions (*saṁskāras)* and desires we are still holding onto due to our nature and our ego. Perhaps what we hold onto is our religious fervor for God, and we think this is a good thing. Or perhaps what we hold onto is our need to help others, to be of service in the world, and we think this is a good thing. The fact is, holding onto any desire or need or belief is ego driven. The Mother says that the nature of the mind is to take a part and call it a whole and exclude all other parts. This is a sign of spiritual incompleteness and immaturity.

Practice: Practice the various *dhyāna kriyās* pertaining to the five sense organs (*pañca-indriyāni),* as taught in *Babaiji's Kriya Yoga* level I and III initiations. Seek inspiration and the opening of the subtle senses. Practice the *Yoga* of the Nine Openings as taught in level III to purify the subconscious attractions through the five senses.

48. *tato mano-javitvaṃ vikaraṇa-bhāvaḥ pradhāna-jayaś-ca*

tataḥ = thence; consequently

manas = mind

javitvam = quickness; speed, swiftness

vikaraṇabhāvaḥ = superphysical sensory capability

pradhāna = originator; primary cause, Nature the most essential part of something; supreme soul; the intellect

jaya = mastery

ca = and

From this comes quickness of the mind, superphysical sensory capability, and mastery over the primary cause.

Mastery over the sense organs (*vikaraṇa*) brings mastery over their corresponding subtle counterparts. *Javitva* is the condition wherein consciousness can quickly move between levels in the mind, from the subconscious to the superconscious. *Pradhāna* is synonymous to *prakṛti or* Nature, in *Samkhya* philosophy, which includes 24 or more elements or principles. Communion (*saṁyama*) with these brings mastery of the principles of nature (*tattvas*).

Once we gain mastery over the sense organs, it is a kind of liberation, for we are free of motivation. The action becomes a thing, free of attachment to the results, therefore free of consequence. When asked for advice, what to do about this or that situation? The Mother invariably answered: "Do whatever you like, it doesn't matter."

Practice: See the invisible hand of the Divine guiding you. Feel yourself to be an instrument of the Divine, without pride, doing your duty as skillfully as possible.

49. *sattva-puruṣa-anyatā-khyāti-mātrasya sarva-bhāva-adhiṣṭhātṛtvaṃ sarva-jñātṛtvaṃ ca*

sattva = being, lightness, beingness, existence

puruṣa = Self

anyatā = distinction; difference

khyātimātra = mere, here, only;

sarva = over all

bhāva = states of being; existence

adhiṣṭhātṛtva = supremacy; literally: "having the quality of standing above or over;" sovereignty, supremacy

sarva = all

jñātṛtva = omniscience literally "the state of being a *jñātṛ* (one who is knowing, intelligent and wise); omniscience

ca = and

By seeing the distinction between the Self and being, [the adept]

gains supremacy over all states [of existence] and omniscience.

After obtaining the powers described in previous verses one may develop omnipotence and omniscience if one gives up the desire for them. This paradox was introduced in verse II.26, wherein uninterrupted discriminative discernment (*viveka-khyātir-aviplavā)* between the Self and the transitory was prescribed as the sole means for attaining the highest, seedless (*nirbīja*) state of non-distinguished cognitive absorption (*asaṁprajñātaḥ samādhi*). By distinguishing the Self from "being": who may exercise omnipotence (*sarva-bhāva-adhiṣṭhātṛtvaṃ)* or omniscience (*sarva-jñātṛtvaṃ),* one leaves behind the latter. To put it succinctly, "when you give it all up, you get it all." Or, "when you become purified enough to acquire the power to move mountains, you no longer desire to move them, so they stay where they are."

Practice: Practice *nirvikalpa samādhi kriyā,* as taught in the Third Level Initiation of *Babaji's Kriya Yoga* level III initiation, until by repeated practice (*abhyāsa),* it becomes fixed within, present during all states. Thereafter, one is guided from within.

50. *tad-vairāgyād-api doṣa-bīja-kṣaye kaivalyam*

tad = that; this

vairāgyāt = because of or due to non-attachment

api = even

doṣa = impediment, detriment, fault, want; obstacle

bīja = seed

kṣaye = in the destruction

kaivalyam = absolute freedom (see IV.34), absolute unity, beatitude, detachment from all other connections; aloneness

Through detachment even towards [the *siddhis* of omniscience and

omnipotence with] the destruction of the seed of this obstacle, there arises absolute freedom.

A thought is an arrow shot at the truth; it can hit a point, but not cover the whole target. But the archer is too well satisfied with his success to ask anything further. The image is perfect for people who imagine they have found the Truth, simply because they have managed to touch one point. That is not enough. One must know all viewpoints and the usefulness of all things. Everything is useful and has its place. There can be no conflicting thoughts. You see the whole without division. There are no choices to be made. There is only a vision of THAT.

"When you are in a condition to receive it, you receive from the Divine the Totality of the relationship you are capable of having; it is neither a share nor a part nor a repetition, but exclusively and uniquely the relationship each one is capable of having with the Divine. Thus, from the psychological point of view, You Alone have this direct relationship with the Divine. One is all alone with the Supreme." (Agenda of the Mother, 8-22-56)

Tirumūlar defines absolute freedom (*kaivalyam)* as union with Śiva, and this requires going beyond distinctions and powers as discussed in the commentary on verse III.49.

> They tarry not in the Pure *māyā* Sphere of Śiva *tattvas,*
> There they but attain the status of Gods,
> But that is a springboard,
> Their Soul reaches farther out to Himself
> And merging in His Union, Self-effacing,
> Themselves become Immaculate Śiva
> They, forsooth, are *śuddha Śaivas.* (TM 1440)

And

> I sought Him in terms of I and You,
> But He that knows not I from You
> Taught me the Truth: "I" indeed is "You,"
> And now I talk not of "I" and "You." (TM 1441)

Like Patañjali, who began by distinguishing beingness (*sattva*) from the Self, Tirumular went beyond into "all one-ness."

Practice: Practice *Nirvikalpa samādhi kriyā,* letting go of all insights and points of view.

51. *sthāny-upanimantraṇe saṅga-smaya-akaraṇaṃ punar-aniṣṭa-prasaṅgāt*

sthāni = well-established, having a place; occupying a high position

upanimantraṇe = invitation, offer;

saṅga = attachment

smaya = smile (with pride); pride, arrogance

akaraṇam = no cause; causeless; absence of action

punar = again

aniṣṭa = undesirable; unwanted, undesirable

prasaṅgāt = because of an association; devotion to, attachment or adherence

[Even] at the invitation of celestial beings [the adept should] not indulge any attachment or pride [because] undesired and renewed lower tendencies [may develop].

This verse refers to a very high and subtle level of consciousness involving interaction with *devas* or celestial beings, for example in a vision, dream, out of the body experience. Such beings, while not existing on the physical plane, may offer all manner of distractions, pleasures and flattery, but throughout the experience the *yogin* should remain in a state of supreme detachment *para-vairgya.* All spiritual experiences prepare us, providing a transition to and a basis for further development. What is necessary is not to indulge in experiences with celestial beings but to maintain an aspiration for progress, and a will for perfection. But often what people really desire are the visions and occult experiences. That for them is concrete. If we are attached to admiration of celestial beings, and we get that experience, we might become complacent. The best part of our being may begin to relax its aspiration for the true goal. Just keep on with it.

Practice: Although celestial beings may not be raining flowers down on you, with a little attention you may notice that you are having spiritual dreams or premonitions, or hearing voices somewhere in your head giving you words of encouragement, or feeling or sensing support around you. Believe in these experiences. These beings exist all around us and with a wide enough consciousness we can become aware of them.

52. *kṣaṇa-tat-kramayoḥ saṃyamād viveka-jaṃ jñānaṃ*

kṣaṇa = moment; an instantaneous moment in time; a measure of time;

tad = its this; that

kramayoḥ = sequence; succession

saṃyamāt = because of or owing to communion

viveka-jaṁ = produced or arising from discrimination,

jñānam = knowledge

There is knowledge born from the arising of discrimination due to communion on the succession of instantaneous moments of time.

Throughout all of one's life we experience one thing after another, the divine purpose of which is to remove the scales from our eyes. As we study the moments of our life in sequence, it may appear that there are two distinct beings within you. One is more real than the other, because it has been given more expression; it is more realized, more conscious of itself, but it stands back, deep below the surface. The other being, the surface personality, a huge collection of thoughts and feelings, does not yet have the power to openly direct you to your destiny, and so may find yourself wandering around in circles, like a blind person.
Practice: By focusing your awareness on single moments you may

discover what is keeping you from realizing your destiny. Look for people or situations in your life, which cause you tension, sap your vitality, or discourage you. Look at what you are willing, or not willing, to sacrifice for Self-realization. Practice the technique of continual bliss (*nityānanda kriyā*) as taught in the *Babaji's Kriya Yoga* level II initiation.

53. *jāti lakṣaṇa deśair-anyatā-anavacchedāt-tulyayos-tataḥ pratipattiḥ*

jāti = category; birth; origination

lakṣaṇa = appearance; mark, sign, symbol, token, characteristic; a favorable sign;

deśaiḥ = with or by the points, regions parts, places or portions

anyatā = distinctions; difference

anavacchedāt = because of being unlimited, not separate, continuous

tulyayoḥ = of the sameness (of two things)

tatas = thus; hence

pratipattiḥ = perception, ascertainment, observation

Hence there is the ascertainment of two similar [things], [owing to the fact that] they are not being limited by differences of origination, markings and place.

Material objects may appear similar, but there is a reality, which lies behind them. One begins to see through similar looking objects by connecting with That which lies behind the distinctions of vital or mental "reality."

As Chapple and Viraj have pointed out: "The traditional reading of Vyasa states a *yogin* is able to tell two identical items apart despite their occupying the same space but at different times. This signifies that all things are in a state of flux. As a variant reading, this *sutra* might refer to the similarity between the *sattva* or unmanifest form of *prakriti* and the *purusa.* For a list of their similarities, see s*amkhya Karika XI.* The key to liberation is to be able to see the difference between these two; this is the highest *siddhi* of *kaivalyam.* This context is borne out by the context before and after this passage. (See III:45 and III:55)".**(12)**

Practice: Practice the *nadi dhyana kriya,* as taught in the *Babaji's Kriya Yoga level I initiation,* to realize the distinctions behind appearances.

54. *tārakaṃ sarva-viṣayaṃ sarvathā-viṣayam-akramaṇ ca-iti viveka-jaṃ jñānam*

tāraka = enabling to cross over, rescuing, liberating, saving

sarva = all

viṣaya = condition

sarvathā = in every way or respect, at all times

viṣayam = object

akrama = without sequence; succession

ca = and

iti = thus; at the end of a clause it also indicates the end of a quotation or saying; "it is said that"

viveka-jaṁ = produced of arising from discrimination,

jñāna = knowledge

And, it is said that, the knowledge born of discrimination is liberating, non-sequential and [inclusive] of all conditions and all times.

The *sūtras* as a whole may be considered as the wisdom wherein one becomes all things and all times regardless of limitations. In the *Tirumantiram* this collective wisdom is referred to as The Path of Knowledge (*jñāna-mārga).*

She is Wisdom subtle,
Of those with intellect subtle,
Behind it is Lord's Wisdom,
That is *Jñāna*;
That Way is the Holy Way,
For those who seek Śiva-State,
That Way is the Holy Way,
For those who seek Śiva-state,
The way of San*-mārga* (*Tam.)* (*jñāna)* is Way True. (TM 1228)

Wisdom is also the fruit of the efforts and experiences, which have preceded it, and may come in stages. Such stages are referred to in the *Tirumantiram* as *carya, kriyā* and *yoga. Carya* (literally "course or motion") is defined in TM verse 1444 as "to adore Siva in love" the path of devotion, of the servitor, leading to *sālokya (Tam.) mukti,* wherein the devotee abides in the sphere of the Lord; *kriyā* is defined as either ritualistic worship or inner sacrificial worship involving the nine orifices of the human body, likened to the nine sacrificial fire pits used in rituals of fire (*yajñas)*; it leads to *saṁipa)(Tam.) mukti,* wherein the devotee is close to the Lord, as his child; *yoga,* joining or union of the soul with the immortal being and consciousness and delight of the Divine: the path of the Lord's friend, leading to *sārūpya (Tamil for svarupa)-mukti.* Herein the devotee attains the form and various insignia of the Lord. This ultimately leads to *sayujya mukti* wherein one attains Oneness with the Supreme Being (see TM verses 1015, 1228-29, 1427, 1477-87, 1507-1513, 1567, 1701, 2679).

Discrimination takes place when we understand what is important in our development and what is a distraction along the way. The supernatural is interesting, but it is not indispensable for Yoga. The Mother suggests that an important part is to be able to get through the lid at the top of the skull, which keeps our consciousness shut into the physical, vital and mental dimensions. There is a cover, which you must get rid of. If you can do this you are ripe for *Yoga.* It is like the opening to the higher mind, a mental opening to the higher realms.

Practice: Practice *kriyā kuṇḍalinī prāṇāyāma,* the higher *cakra kriyās, prāṇāyāmas* and *mantras,* and the *samādhi kriyās,* as taught in *Babaji's Kriya Yoga* level III initiation, to open the higher mind and to the wisdom born of discernment.

55. *sattva-puruṣayoḥ śuddhi-sāmye kaivalyam-iti*

sattva = being; beingness

puruṣayoḥ = of the the Self

śuddhi = purity

sāmya = in, at, to or concerning equality, evenness, sameness

kaivalyam = aloneness; isolation; absolute freedom

In the sameness of purity between beingness and the Self, there is absolute freedom.

As in the commentary on verse III.50, when the subtlest part of one's being, consciousness (*citta),* becomes completely free of all attachments (*rāgāḥ)* and aversions (*dveṣāḥ),* it merges with the Self. Or as Tirumūlar would put it "*Jīva* becomes Śiva." The removal of the afflictions (*kleśas)* from the mind by purification was discussed in verse II.3 and II.10. Like a lake, in which the sediment drops to the bottom, when the habit of identifying with the movements within consciousness subsides, one becomes transparent. Oneness with the Supreme Being is realized.

The Mother describes what happens when Absolute Freedom or Aloneness is established. "When there is equality in purity between one's being and the Self, then it all happens spontaneously. It just happens and it's another way of being. Then nothing will have the power to make one fall back into the old movement. And whether you are walking around or washing up, nothing shakes you from That. All you see is That - Consciousness. It is a Consciousness, a Presence. And all, is there together, the Power, the Presence, the Consciousness, that joy and Love. And all of that together almost gives the impression of a Form, that Vibration of a Form and yet no form."

<u>Practice</u>: Remember this quote: "One must never go back; one must

always go forward. The curves of life will take us this way and that, we must go straight beyond. Do not hold grudges. All sincere feelings should remain. Do not decide anything mentally. Learn to be immobile, silent and let the Lord speak through you. Even in difficult situations depend on your Faith in the Lord to do what's best, and say, "All right, let's see what happens!" "The less one explains, the less one plans, the better - always, always."(13)

Chapter 4: KAIVALYA PĀDA

This concluding chapter brings us to the end of our quest: absolute freedom (*kaivalya),* or what Sri Aurobindo called "Absolute Unity".**(1)** It reminds us of the cardinal teaching of Jesus: "Be ye perfect, even as your Father in Heaven is perfect," and "Ye are Gods, and all of you are children of the most High" (Psalms lxxxii, 6; quoted by Jesus John x.34). This teaching has been overshadowed by the mistaken dogma that Jesus was "the only begotten son God."

The curious opposition between the "spirit and the flesh," found in so many traditions, East and West alike, has found itself into most of the previous commentaries on the *Sūtras.* Even while there is the recognition that the union (*yoga)* between the Self (*puruṣa)* and Nature (*prakṛti*) is the final attainment, the bias of these commentators against Nature, particularly, human nature, has prevented them from realizing the great potential for Self-realization to transform Nature. It is as if they have assumed that the known laws of Nature are immutable. They have for the most part concluded, that the final state of Self-realization, *kaivalya* must necessarily involve a departure of the realized soul from the physical plane. Divorce between the spirit and flesh again! Sri Aurobindo in his works, *The Divine Life,* and *The Synthesis of Yoga,***(2)** however, has indicated the potential for a *supramental descent,* which would transform Nature, as we ordinarily know it.

Patañjali has already told us in verse I.3 that "the Seer abides in his or her own true form (*svarūpa*)." The individual soul (*jiva)* assumes, by expansion, its true nature or form (*Śiva).* In other words, there is a union (*Yoga)* of *puruṣa* as pure Consciousness (*cit)* with Nature (*prakṛti).* As indicated in verse IV.2, this union may involve a radical transformation at various levels. The ordinary human nature, previously motivated only by the constituent forces of nature (*guṇas*), is replaced by a higher nature (*svarūpa*), literally, one's own essential or true nature. There are many references to one's own true form or Nature (*svarūpa*) in the literature of the Tamil *Yoga Siddhas.* Tirumūlar referred to it as "self-illuminating manifestness" in dozens of verses (TM 1486, 2441, 2474, 2478-84, 2491, 2496, 2532,

2538, 2566, 2574, 2655, 2675, 2828-29, 2834-46, 2855-64). The numerous parallels between the *Sūtras* and the *Tirumantiram*, as shown in the introduction to this commentary, include a similar conception of final attainment, *kaivalya*. By comparing their conceptions in this final chapter, our own destination, and hence, our path, will become much clearer.

The term *siddhānta* is the final end of perfection or accomplishment for the *Śaivite*. A *siddha* is therefore one who manifests *siddhi* or perfection or attainments. "I am the Supreme One," says the *Vedāntin*; whereas, "I shall become the Supreme One" says the *Siddhāntin*. While, in one sense, *kaivalya* refers to the *yogin's* final attainment, once reached, it also marks the beginning of unlimited possibilities. Other commentators have missed this essential point. For example, Feuerstein has argued that because of the philosophical dualism advocated by the *Sutras, kaivalya* necessitates one's non-involvement in the world when one reaches the highest state of cognitive absorption, *asaṁprajñātaḥ samādhi*. Not even the state of the *jivan mukta* or living, as a liberated soul is possible in such a strictly dualistic philosophical framework.**(3)** But, *Kaivalya*, understood not as merely an end, but also a beginning, is therefore, completely synonymous with the state of a *siddha*, who has realized Absolute Unity with the Supreme Being in the spiritual plane of existence, by self-surrender(*sva- praṇidhānam)*, allowing the Supreme Being (*Īśvara)* to descend within oneself at all levels. This brings about an integrated transformation of human nature, including the intellect, mental, vital and physical. Only such an all-encompassing transformation merits recognition with the term "perfection." To be spiritually awakened in a diseased body, neurotic mind, or disturbed vital, is not perfection.

The *siddhas* were not fakirs or jugglers, manifesting accomplishments (*siddhis)* or divine powers for their own sake, nor were the *siddhis* mere amusements, to be discarded as one approached the highest levels of Self-realization. This is the unfortunate image, which many commentators have mistakenly attributed to the *siddhas*. The numerous powers described in the previous chapter are stepping stones, or in many cases, by products of a process which leads to complete and absolute union (*yoga-parama)* with the Lord (*Īśvara)*. In becoming "perfect," manifesting all of the powers of the Divine, they became *siddhas*. Whether the *siddha* continues to manifest on the physical plane or not is of no importance. If the *siddha* does, it is only to be instrumental in the awakening and transformation of the human race. If they leave, it is not because they are forced to leave by a degeneration of the human organism.

In *pāda* 4, Patañjali sets the stage for this final level of Self-realization, which, in reality, is never "final." How could one limit the Divine or his creation? One who is by definition, limitless! The final *pāda*, the fifth, is yet to be written, by all of us.

1. *janma-oṣadhi-mantra-tapaḥ-samādhi-jāḥ siddhyayaḥ*

janman = birth; existence

oṣadhi = medicinal herb; medicine. From *osa,* meaning light containing, and referring probably to the photosynthesis of plants.

mantra = literally "protection of the mind;" sacred text or speech; incantation; a mystical verse; "instrument of thought." From *manas (*mind) and *tara* (protection).

tapas = intense practice; glowing, straightening by fire; "the burning away of the burden of one's *karma.*"

samādhi = cognitive absorption

jāḥ = born; arisen

siddhayaḥ = powers; perfection, attainment; accomplishment

The powers are the result of birth, herbs, *mantras,* intense practice, and cognitive absorption.

Some may argue that because Patañjali did not speak of *kuṇḍalinī* or *śakti*; he had no knowledge of *tantra.* They ignore this verse, and others, where he speaks of worship of the Lord (*īśvara,* I.24 and II.1). They also perhaps forget the broader meaning of *kuṇḍalinī,* which is our potential power and consciousness. While Patañjali does not refer to it by name, nor with the symbolism used by the practitioners of *tantra (tantrikas),* the entire third *pāda* of the *Sūtras* is a description of what can only be termed our "potential power and consciousness." The succinct writing style of the *Sūtras* and perhaps an intention by Patañjali to present *yoga* as a philosophy shorn of sectarian symbols, iconography or beliefs, may account for the absence of traditional *tantric* terminology. Even the many verses in the third *pāda* of the *Sūtras* which describe the application of communion (*saṁyama)* on a particular object or idea, refer to what is essentially a *tantric* practice, the union or concentration of form with energy (*śakti)* to realize one's potential.

Often where there is what can be interpreted in retrospect as a "decay" or excess in the implementation of a sacred ideology, other contemporaries have responded by instigating reform. Take the example of the Protestant Reform movement that had simplified religious worship in reaction to the decadence of Christianity beginning in the 15th century. Within religious practice and belief, in moments of ferment and exchange between different sects one can find many examples of spiritual syncretism such as Sikhism, Sufism, Kashmiri Saivism and Hindu Tantra. Patañjali's Kriya Yoga as we know it today could have been born from a kind of syncretism, reformation, or a combination of other complex elements.

Aside from communion *(saṁyama)* the power (*śakti)* described at length in the third *pāda* of the *Sūtras* may develop as a result of powers with which one is born (*jāti*), or which may have been developed in a previous birth. Some herbal formulas (*oṣadhi)* may also induce special powers like clairvoyance (*ādarśa*) or prophecy (precognition). The practice of *mantras* are specific sound formulas, in many cases used in conjunction with ritual geometric symbols (*yantras*) to bring about particular results. These powers may also develop as a result of intensive practice of meditation for prolonged periods (*tapas)* or manifest as a result of entering into cognitive absorption (*samādhi*). Such powers may be used to bring about particular results. For example, in the 1940's, a well known ascetic (*tapasvin)* Prasananda Guru sat next to the *Brahmanur Kali Koyil* near Kanadukatan, Tamil Nadu, without moving for 48 days, in order to end a severe drought. On the 48th day rain began to pour and there has never been a problem with drought since then, in that region. The *tantric* traditions are full of such esoteric knowledge. The entire fourth chapter (*tantra*) of the Tirumaniram is devoted to *mantras and yantras.*

Practice: Set aside extended periods for intensive practice; become initiated into the *mantras* correctly as in *Babaji's Kriya Yoga* level II initiation. Practice these *mantras* extensively; envision the circumstances of your next birth and cultivate the prerequisites in this one. Use medicinal herbs to increase balance, health and vitality.

2. *jāty-antara-pariṇāmaḥ prakṛty-āpūrāt*

jāti-antara = into another species, from *jāti:* birth, and *antara:* different

pariṇāma = change, alteration, evolution, transformation

prakṛti = Nature

āpūrāt = because of, due to, excess, abundance; filling up, making full; vast possibilities

The transformation into another species [is due to] the vast possibilities inherent in Nature.

This aphorism, in conjunction with the previous verse, informs us not only of the possibility but also the likelihood, that the human species as it is now constituted, will evolve into something new, with perhaps as yet undreamed of capabilities. It is a remarkable aphorism given the fact that for the most part, the *Sūtras* in particular, and the traditional texts of *Yoga* in general, speak only of possible attainments of higher states of consciousness for individuals only, as a result of their diligent application of the methods and processes of *yoga.* The collective mutation of the human species is rarely indicated. Sri Aurobindo's *The Divine Life* and Ramalinga Swamigal's *Thiruvarulpa* (Divine Song of Grace) are relatively modern, and notable exceptions.**(4,5)** Both of them experienced a profound transformation at the cellular level of their physical existence and both elaborated on a vision that all humanity could one day undergo such a divine transformation. One cannot, therefore, assume that the higher states of *samādhi* invariably lead to only more rarefied states of human existence, increasingly spiritual, and less and less to do with the gross material body, with all of its suffering and drama. How prescient and remarkable it is to find such a statement here, near the beginning of the last *pāda* of the *Sūtras.* It is as if to announce that as *yogins* we labor not simply for our own individual salvation, but for a new humanity, preferably one which will manifest the divine qualities indicated in verses III.45 and III.46. These include beauty, grace strength, extraordinary endurability and invulnerability of its function.

Among the few *yogins* in modern times who have not only appreciated this possibility of a new human species, but who have greatly elaborated this vision and labored for its birth are Sri Aurobindo and the Mother. See Sri Aurobindo's "The Divine Life," "The Synthesis of Yoga," and "Savitri," as well as the Mother's "Agenda," for more on this next evolutionary step.**(6,7)** With regards to this, mention may also be made to the prediction by Yogananda's guru, Sri Yukteswar that by the year 4000, telepathy would be the common form of communication between humans.

The object of Sri Aurobindo's *Yoga* was "to bring down the supramental consciousness on earth, to fix it steady in a collective group of people creating a new race (not a race of supermen) but a race of people with the principles of the supramental consciousness (laws of wisdom), directing the inner individual and collective lives. That force would have to be accepted individual after individual according to their preparation and would establish a supramental consciousness in the physical world, which would create a nucleus for its own expansion. The new consciousness would affect all peoples. They would feel a greater Light and Power, and it would eventually increase their possibilities."**(8)**

To be ready for such a force the mind must be prepared. A mind must be free of mental concepts and activity. It is only in a silent quiet mind that the greater force can be received and work can be accomplished on the system without too much reaction and resistance.

Practice: Imagine you are in Perfect Unity with the Supreme Consciousness, pull yourself into an unshakeable concentration on That. Live in That minute-to-minute. When you notice a thought, feeling or an old habit trying to pull you out of That, refuse. Step back into the support of that silent, still, luminosity.

3. *nimittam-aprayojakaṃ prakṛtīnāṃ varaṇa-bhedas-tu tataḥ kṣetrikavat*

nimittam = incidental cause; motive; ground; reason

aprayojakam = not causing or effecting; not initiating

prakṛtīnāṁ = manifestations of Nature; here: natural evolution

varaṇa = surrounding; enclosing obstacles

bhedaḥ = separation; division; distinction

tu = but

tatas = from that; hence

kṣetrikavat = like a farmer; like the owner of a field

Incidental events do not [directly] cause natural evolution, but remove the obstacles as a farmer [removes the obstacles in a water course running to his field].

This verse is related to the previous verse IV.2 and describes how Nature manifests, not just as it pertains to individual human beings. The wider implication is that the individual can affect the course of Nature. We impact not only ourselves, but our environment and others socially. Modern theories of deep ecology elaborate on this message, well known to initiates dedicated to *Babaji's Kriya Yoga Pledge*: which says in sum that: "We practice yoga not only for our own benefit, but for the benefit of everyone." It also reminds us of Sri Aurobindo's reply to an appeal that he return to lead the Indian independence movement. He said that what was needed was "not a revolt against the British Government, which anyone could easily manage...(but) a revolt against the whole of universal Nature."**(9)**

The Mother says that one cannot make an effort or try to make it happen, and no intellectual activity is necessary. It is something one must become, something one must be and live. The work is done slowly, like a chick is formed in an egg. You do not know what is going on inside the shell. Inside you feel pushing and feeling pressure and yet there are no results. Then all at once, everything bursts open and everything is done. Everything changes. Your life completely changes existence. You just have to keep at it. Perhaps even events, which appear to cause chaos and upheaval and destruction are simply Nature's way of removing the obstacles, the resistance in the way.**(10)**

Practice: Contemplate the aphorism: "God is infinite possibility. Therefore Truth is never at rest."

4. *nirmāṇa-cittāny-asmitā-mātrāt*

nirmāṇa = creating, making forming, fabricating

citta = consciousness; hence, in this context *nirmāṇa-citta* can mean "individualized" consciousness

asmitā = egoism; "I-am-ness"

mātrāt = limitation; only

The individualized consciousness only [arises] from the limitation of egoism.

In verse II.3 Patañjali listed egoism (*asmitā*), as one of the five causes of affliction (*pañca-upakleśas*) which stand in the way of realization of cognitive absorption (*samādhi*). In II.6, Patañjali defined egoism as "the identification of the Seer, with that of the instrument of seeing (the body-mind)" *(dṛg-darśana-śaktyor-eka-ātmatā-iva-asmitā).* J.W. Hauer (1958)**(11)** has shown that *nirmāṇa-citta* can denote "individualized consciousness;" that is, the part of one's consciousness which is involved in phenomena, such as is experienced as sense objects, thoughts and emotions. This is distinct from what might be called the consciousness at the core of our being, the Self, which stands back as it were, as a witness. In this *sūtra* Patañjali indicates that this individualized consciousness (*nirmāṇa-citta*) originates at that point in Nature's (*prakṛti's*) process of transforming from potentiality to actuality where the subject separates from the object. The point is termed, "the limitation of egoism" *(asmitā-mātra)*. A division occurs between subject and object at this point. In *Sāṁkhya* philosophy this is known as the "I-maker" (*ahaṁkāra*). So the problem of individuation, with all its attendant suffering, has at its origin, a principle in Nature (*prakṛti*). In other words, our suffering originates not outside ourselves, but in our perspective on the manifestations of Nature. To overcome suffering we must change our perspective. It is the *yogin's* task to overcome this limitation of ego by the cultivation of a higher Self consciousness.

We all want to be unique, special personalities that "do" special things in the world. We think we need our senses sharp and our minds full of information in order to make a mark on the world. Our ego strengthens our statement of who we are, and our need to be someone strengthens our ego. While we remain on the level of the senses we see who we are in terms of how others see us to be. We give our individuality and our individual consciousness an independent reality when we organise everything into little bundles with our imagination.

Practice: Detach from the "I" thought. Allow your *mantra* to be substituted for the "I" thought and all that is attached to it. Bear all external activities on the surface of your Being.

5. *pravṛtti-bhede prayojakaṃ cittam-ekam-anekeṣām*

pravṛtti = activities, moving onward, cognition

bhede = different; distinction

prayojakaṁ = director; initiator

cittam = consciousness; mind

ekam = one

anekeṣāṁ = of the many

[Although there is individualized consciousness] in different activities, the initiator is the one consciousness of the many other [individualized consciousnesses].

One consciousness (*cittam-ekam)* pervades all of Nature's manifestation. The principle of egoism individualizes it, however, and creates the artificial impression of division between subject and object. By tracing consciousness back to its root, this Oneness can be apprehended, and the limitation of egoism surpassed.

Although our personalities may be unique, at the core of our being we are the same: "one without a second." When we begin to understand that who we are is the same as who everyone else is, and understand how intimately we are all connected, all we can feel is deep humility and awe. Once we discover who we are, we begin to release our hold on our need for a limited individual self.

Practice: Practice being conscious of what is conscious.

6. *tatra dhyāna-jam-anāśayam*

tatra = there

dhyānajam = evolved through, arises or born from meditation

anāśayam = without residue; here implying "free from subconscious deposits"

There, [what] arises from meditation is without residue.

After describing how consciousness becomes individualized, Patañjali reminds us that meditation *(dhyāna)* provides a means to become free of deposits in the subconscious. These deposits we were told, in I.24, are the fruit of our action (*karma-vipāka)*, and their removal is the first objective of *Yoga* (see verse I.2). The habitual movements or fluctuations of consciousness arising within consciousness (*citta-vṛttiḥ)* are rooted in these subconscious deposits. As these deposits are gradually removed one remains more and more as the Seer. (see verse I.3)

Practice: The *śuddhi dhyāna kriyā* and techniques related to the Nine Openings of the body taught in the *Babaji's Kriya Yoga* level III initiation. Contemplate Sri Aurobindo's words: "In the calm mind, it is the substance of the mental being that is still, so still that nothing disturbs it. If thoughts or activities come, they do not rise at all out of the mind, but they come from outside and cross the mind as a flight of birds crosses the sky in a windless air. It passes, disturbs nothing, leaving no trace. Even if a thousand images or the most violent events pass across it, the calm stillness remains as if the very texture of the mind were a substance of eternal and indestructible peace. A mind that has achieved this calmness can begin to act, even intensely and powerfully, but it will keep its fundamental stillness - originating nothing from itself but receiving from Above and giving it a mental form without adding anything of its own, calmly, dispassionately, though with the joy of the Truth and the happy power and light of its passage."**(12)**

7. *karma-aśukla-akṛṣṇaṃ yoginnnas-trividham-itareṣām*

karma = action

aśukla = not white; pure, stainless

akṛṣṇa = not black or dark

yoginnnas = the Yogin; one who has *Yoga*

trividham = threefold

itareṣha = of others.

The *karma* of the *yogin* is neither white nor black; [but the *karma* of] others is threefold.

Here, *karma* refers not only to good and bad, but to all kinds of categories and differentiations. *Karma* is traditionally considered to be of three types: good, bad and mixed. Good *karma* are actions which bring one closer to the goal of *samādhi*; bad *karma* keeps one in the noose of *saṁskāra* with all of its suffering; mixed implies actions which bring both happiness and suffering. Of course too much of happiness producing *karma* may eventually create suffering. For example, to feed someone in need indefinitely will eventually lead to a situation where not only will they lose their independence, but they will also suffer much resentment. For the accomplished *yogin*, one established in *para-vairagya* (supreme detachment) there is no more interest in seeking happiness or avoiding suffering. That duality based, desire driven attitude is seen as a trap of the ego based consciousness. When the accomplished *yogin* reaches non-distinguished cognitive absorption (*asaṁprajñātaḥ samādhi*), he or she no longer creates any more subconscious impressions (*saṁskāra* or *vāsanā*). So the yogin creates no new roots for any future *karma*. However, until then, the *yogin* in development must be vigilant with regards to desires and continue to practice intensively (see verse II.2) in order to remove the deposit roots of karma.

For an advanced *yogin,* even actions directed toward them from others can be deflected. It is the mind, which judges actions good, bad or indifferent and reacts against them, reaping the results. The *yogin* simply witnesses actions, without judgment and with detachment (*vairāgya).*

Practice: Be a witness to all things without judgment. Perform actions selflessly, after reflection, without attachment to the results. Maintain equanimity in success or failure, praise or blame, loss or gain, good things and bad things. Be vigilant in noticing and rejecting ego-based motivations.

8. *tatas-tad-vipāka-anuguṇānām-eva-abhivyaktir-vāsanām*

tatas = hence

tad = this or that

eva = thus, only

vipāka = fruition

anuguṇānām = having similar qualitiesfavorable condition

eva = alone

abhivyaktir = manifestation, distinction

vāsanānām = subconscious impressions; the impression of anything remaining in the mind; knowledge derived from memory

Hence, only those subconscious impressions for which there are favorable conditions for producing their fruits, will manifest.

This verse extends verse II.12 and II.13, which explain how the fruition (*vipāa)* of subconscious deposits (*saṁskāra)* takes place, often waiting for the appropriate birth or circumstances corresponding to the *saṁskāra*. There is almost always a correspondence between our actions (*karma)* and subconscious deposits (*saṁskāra)*. The exception occurs when there is a conscious volition to break out of this vicious circle of subconscious habit and karma laden action. The exercise of one's conscious volition can be considered as a *sādhana* or "remembrance of who one truly is and what one is not, and can manifest through all those disciplines of yoga," as described in the second *pāda,* including the cultivation of the opposites to negative thoughts.

One problem, which this implies, is that our subconscious impressions are so easily distorted by our judgments and prejudices, beliefs and fears, that we do not even see the consequences clearly before acting. We create more *karma* by working things out in our minds, with a distorted vision.

Practice: In each situation, still the mind, and allow yourself to see the Truth. Avoid reacting immediately on subconscious impressions.

9. *jāti-deśa-kāla-vyavahitānām-apy-ānantaryaṃ smṛti-saṃskārayor-eka-rūpatvāt*

jāti = class or species; life state, birth

deśa = space; place

kāla = time

vyavahitānām = concealedseparated

api = though, even

ānantaryam = link, immediate sequence or succession

smṛti = memory

saṃskārayor = subconscious impressions

ekarūpatvāt = because of the uniformity; one form, one kind,

As memory and residual subsconscious impressions are of one form, there is a link even [with] the separation of birth, place, time.

In other words, "past actions, even if not remembered, continue to affect present actions".**(13)** Karma leaves impressions in individualized consciousness. Each one's subconscious is personalized as a result of the uniformity (*ekarūpatvāt)* between memory (*smṛti)* and the subconscious impressions (*saṁskāras).* These are carried over to the future, so each individual's actions are a function of the *karma* driven subconscious impressions, rather than being determined by some collective reservoir of impression common to all humanity. These impressions are cumulative and relative in their force and influence. Some subconscious impressions, such as a tendency to easily become angry, may be neutralized by others such as a tendency to forgive others. Here Patañjali wants to emphasize that it is our accumulated subconscious impressions (*saṁskāra),* which determine our actions (*karma),* and that this personalized set of *saṁskāras* may express itself in different time periods, settings and even existences (that is future births or as another species).

Practice: Practice being a witness, seeing events with detachment, and accept the working out of your karma with equanimity.

10. *tāsām-anāditvaṃ ca-āśiso nityatvāt*

tāsām = of these [impressions]

anāditvam = beginninglessness; the state of having no beginning

ca = and

āśisaḥ = asking for, prayer, wish, desire, benediction; a boon with permanent character sure fulfillment

nityatvāt = because of eternality, continuance

These [impressions] are beginningless, because desires are eternal.

Mother Nature's fundamental urge to live, to grow, to express itself through desire has as a consequence an endless, and therefore, beginingless number of forms and creations, including these subconscious impressions (*saṁskāras)* recorded in the memory (*smṛtiḥ).* Desire includes the clinging to life. See *sutras* II.3 and II.9, which mentioned it as one of the five afflictions (*kleśas).* One of the strongest primary identifications we have is with the body. And we are born with a very strong attachment to life in that body. Until we realize that we are not the body, this primary will to live causes us to fear death.

Practice: Remember: "Abide in Me (*Babaji*) and allow the transformation of these impressions to proceed." Always be patient with yourself.

11. *hetu-phala-āśraya-ālambanaiḥ saṃgṛhītatvād-eṣām-abhāve tad-abhāvaḥ*

hetu = cause

phala = fruit; result; effect

āśraya = correspondence; basis; that on which anything depends; dependence

ālambanaiḥ = by or with the supports or basis

saṃgṛhītatvāt = because, due to or owing to that which is seized, grasped, caught, gathered

eṣāṁ = of these or those

abhāve = in, on, at or concerning the non-becoming disappearance; absence

tat = that or this

abhāvaḥ = non-becoming disappear; absence

The impressions being held together by cause, effect, basis and support, they disappear with the disappearance of these four.

Here cause (*hetu)* refers to the primary cause of suffering cited in verses II.4 which is ignorance (*avidyā,* i.e. confusing the Self with the non-Self), and which gives rise to the other afflictions: ego (*asmitā),* attachment, aversion (*dveṣa)* and the desire for existence (*abhiniveṣaḥ)* (see II.3 to II.9) Effect or fruit (*phala)* refers to the fruition of cause or actions (*karma,* see IV.8). Basis (*ālambana)* refers to the memory (*smṛtiḥ*), or that type of movement of consciousness existing as a personal field in each person (see verse IV.9). Support (*āśraya)* refers to the stimulus, whether it be objective (sense based) or subjective, which is presented to consciousness.

Here Patañjali tells us that while we cannot remove the subconscious impressions (*saṁskāras)* directly, by weakening our involvement in, or identification with, these four factors of cause, effect, basis and support which hold the *saṁskāras* together, they will gradually disappear. Exactly how we may detach from this involvement is the process of Y*oga* as discussed elsewhere (for example, see verses II.2 and II.11)

Practice: Intensely and continuously practice self study (*svādhyāya),* detachment (*vairāgya),* and surrender (*praṇidhāna).*

12. *atīta-anāgataṃ sva-rūpato' sty-adhva-bhedād-dharmāṇām*

atīta = past

anāgatam = future; yet to come

svarūpataḥ = in reality, from one's own form; according to one's own form

a*sti* = [it] exists, is

adhva = path, road, way, course; flow

bhedāt = because of the difference, distinction or separation *dharmāṇām* = of the forms, characteristics, essential qualities, virtues

The past and future exist in the real form of objects which manifest due to differences in the flow of forms [produced by Nature].

Past and future are real. Over time, Nature, the primary substance of all creation (*prakṛti),* is modified and individual forms evolve from pure potentiality to manifestation and then back again to pure potentiality. The past includes all those forms, which were once manifested, and have returned to the realm of pure potentiality. The future includes all possible forms, yet to be manifested.

One can observe the past and future existing very practically in the form of spiritual writings. The same One Consciousness who wrote these writings years ago will also be the same Consciousness who will read these writings in years to come. The same Consciousness which existed in the past, in all various forms, exists today in a similar or different form and will exist in the future in other forms.

Practice: Contemplate the thought of the individual Self as a drop in the Ocean.

13. *te vyakta-sūkṣmā guṇa-ātmānaḥ*

te = these [forms]

vyakta = manifest

sūkṣmā = subtle

guṇâtmānaḥ = constituent forces of nature

These [forms] have manifest and subtle constituent forces of Nature.

The forms of Nature *(prakṛti)* may be subtle (*sūkṣma)* or manifested (*vyaktaḥ),* as discussed in verse I.16 and I.19. Whether subtle or material they are composed of the constituent forces, or moods, of nature (*guṇas*); that is, the forces of action (*rajas* or mutation), inertia (*tamas or* statis) and equilibrium (*sattva or* sentience).

Something like a clod of clay is manifest if it is present or visible. As a pot, which existed in the past or will exist in the future, it is subtle. The five elements (*pañca-bhūta)* and the "I-sense" are subtle, but the organs of sense, the organs of action and the mind are manifest.

Practice: Reflect upon how each form is controlled by these three forces.

14. *pariṇāma-ekatvād vastu-tattvam*

pariṇāma = transformation

ekatvāt = because of the oneness or uniformity

vastu = thing; object

tattvam = suchness; reality; thatness, essence

From the oneness of transformation, there is the reality of an object.

While Nature (*prakṛti)* is continually changing, it appears to have a static reality whenever a primary constituent force repeats itself, from one moment to the next. Patañjali explains the appearance of permanency in things by referring to the repeating patterns in the three primary modes of Nature's force (*tri-guṇas).* Unlike *Vedāntic* philosophy, which emphasized the illusion (*māyā)* of the world, both the *Sāṁkhya* based *Sūtras* and the *Tirumantiram* emphasize the reality of things as Nature manifesting according to the 24 or more principles (*tattvas),* including these *guṇas.*

Sattvic is *Guṇa* in the Waking State,
Rajas in Dream State,
Tamas in Deep Sleep State,
Nirguṇa, that other three *Guṇas* destroys,
Is attribute of *Turiya* State Pure. (TM 2296)

Though different, the three act in unison and produce change. They are present in all changes. For example, in the knowledge of sound, there must be potentiality, activity and perceptibility. When we observe the objects of the world from a balanced spiritual perspective, we may distinguish things, which are wholesome and edifying from those, which are disturbing and hence fit to be discarded. Suffering and objects which create suffering, are mutable and fit to be discarded. What is permanent, pure, alive and free is edifying and wholesome. One must go through this process of discrimination so long as one seeks spiritual freedom. However, once attained, it is not necessary to look at the objects of this world from such a spiritual perspective, discarding some things. What remains after the ultimate goal is attained, "the Seer abides in his true nature" (verse I.3) is beyond the comprehension of ordinary individualized consciousness.

Practice: Practice the *inai rūpa dhyāna kriyā* (literally, "meditation of moving form" *kriyā*), and *pūrṇa bhāva indriya dhyāna kriyā* (literally, "meditation on emotion-filled senses" *kriyā*) as taught in *Babaji's Kriya Yoga* level I initiation and observe each of these forces of nature.

15. *vastu-sāmye citta-bhedāt-tayor-vibhaktaḥ panthāḥ*

vastu = object

sāmye = in or concerning equality; sameness, same

citta = consciousness; mind

bhedāt = due to difference, distinction, separations; multiplicity

tayoh = of, in or concerning both these; each; their

vibhaktaḥ = divided, distributed, separated, may vary

panthāh = path, way, road, course

Due to multiplicity of consciousness, the way of [perception] of even the same objects may vary.

In verse IV.4 Patañjali explained how consciousness (*citta*) becomes individualized due to ego (*āsmita*). As a consequence, everyone has an individualized consciousness, and so perceptions of the same object may vary from one person to another. Perception is usually colored by desire, in particular, and by subconscious impressions in general. One could consider the objects and individual consciousness as existing on different levels of existence. The level of existence of the object was explained in the previous three verses.

Until we are able to see without the involvement of the ego, we will not be able to perceive the essential reality within things. In ordinary consciousness we know things only by the intellect, the mind, and the senses, and we know them only through their outward manifestation, results and inferences.

Practice: Listen to the intuition in your observances. See beyond the obvious in every situation. Practice unconditional love with others. It's the quickest way to become attuned to the essential reality within all things.

16. *na ca-eka-citta-tantraṃ vastu tad-apramāṇakaṃ tadā kiṃ syāt*

na = not

ca = and

eka = one

citta = consciousness; mind

tantram = thread, essential part, main point, teaching; here: dependent

vastu = object

tad = that, this

apramāṇakam = not proven or demonstrated; here: perceived

tadā = then

kiṃ = what

syāt = becomes

Nor does an object's existence depend upon a single consciousness, for if it did, what would become of that object when that consciousness did not perceive it?

Here Patañjali points to the distinction between each sense object, the five sense organs (*buddhīndriyāṇi* or *jñānendryāṇi)* of the ears, eyes, nose, skin and tongue that may apprehend it and the five elements (*pañca-bhūta)* of earth, water, fire, air and ether, by which sensation is possible. The absence of the sense organs or sense elements does not annul the existence of the sense object. In other words, all objects are the product of the *gunas* of *prakriti* and are not the product of a single mind.

Practice: Practice using the *pūrṇa bhāva indriya dhyāna kriyā* (literally, "meditation on emotion-filled senses" *kriyā),* as taught in the Babaji's *Kriya Yoga* level I initiation, reflecting upon the distinction between objects, the sense elements and the sense organs.

17. *tad-uparāga-apekṣitvāc-cittasya vastu jñāta-ajñātam*

tad = that

uparāga = coloring; dying, darkening

apekṣitvāt = because of or due to anticipation, expectation; wished, looked for; the state of requiring or depending upon

cittasya = of consciousness or mind

vastu = object

jñāta = known

ajñāta = unknown

An object is known or unknown dependent on [upon] whether or not the consciousness gets colored by it.

We recognize objects because in our memory there is a subconscious deposit associated with a previous experience with such an object.

Patañjali calls this the coloring of consciousness. It is a metaphor for the way we remember.

The Self is the ultimate subject, so it is always superior to all objects of consciousness (*uparāga-cittasya)*. One can only be aware because the movements arising within consciousness are always perceived by the Self. The mind cannot be aware of the Self. Only the Self, or superior (*prabhu)*, can be aware of what occurs within consciousness. When Consciousness becomes conscious of the pure Self, the fundamental background, or root-consciousness, we call this Self-Realization.

Practice: Notice how recognition depends upon memory (*smṛti)*. When you see things as if for the first time, pure consciousness comes to the foreground. Be conscious of what is conscious.

18. *sadā jñātās-citta-vṛttayas-tat-prabhoḥ puruṣasya-apariṇāmitvāt*

sadā = always

jñātaḥ = known

citta = consciousness; mind

vṛttayaḥ = modifications; fluctuations

tat = that; this

prabhoḥ = Superior; master

puruṣasya = of the Self

apariṇāmitvāt = because of or due to the changelessness

The fluctuations of consciousness are always known, because of the changelessness of the Self, [who is] master.

The movements within the individual consciousness (*citta-vṛttayaḥ)* can only be perceived by that which witnesses them, the fundamental background of root-consciousness, which is Stillness, the Self. As one stands back as a witness, one may realize that all actions of the forces of nature are part of a universal working, and actions or events are not necessarily a result of one's conscious action or personality. The changeless Self may be working events through you and making use of something in your nature. But you are generally not conscious of this.

Practice: Contemplate the evolution of life and the working out of all its myriad possibilities.

19. *na tat-sva-ābhāsaṃ dṛśyatvāt*

na = not

tat = that [consciousness]

svābhāsaṁ = self-luminosity; own light

dṛśyatvāt = because being seen; the nature of being seen [object]

That [fluctuations of consciousness] are not self-luminous because they are seen [objects].

Consciousness (*citta*) is an object to the Self, or Seer, and it is in Light of the Self that consciousness is able to perceive. Individual consciousness reflects the Light of the Self. Without the Self, consciousness could not perceive external objects. There cannot be a seer of a Seer. That is why the Seer is self-luminous. This expresses with great similarity the pan-Tibetan Buddhist description of the luminosity of the mind, which is called the *sambhogakaya* or enjoyment body.**(14)**

The mind is not self-luminous either, because it is knowable. That which is knowable is very different from the Knower. Modifications of the mind like attachment, fear, anger, etc. thus become objects or knowables. Only pure subject, the Seer, is capable of being Self-luminous.

The Seer is the Luminous Infinite, the essence hiding behind the individual consciousness with all of its fluctuations, and its instrument, the mind.

Practice: Lie down and allow the body to be relaxed, and very still. Imagine being engulfed in white light. Imagine all of the cells of the body becoming diffused with this light and conscious of their eternity.

20. *eka-samaye ca-ubhaya-anavadhāraṇam*

eka = one and the same

samaye = time; circumstance, instance, occasion

ca = and

ubhaya = both

anavadhāraṇam = non discernment; non perception

Consequently, consciousness cannot perceive both [subject and object] simultaneously.

Consciousness (*citta)* can perceive objects (*vastu),* but it cannot at the same time become aware of itself. Only the higher Self can perceive consciousness and its modifications (*citta-vṛttiḥ).* The Self is incapable of becoming the object of awareness of any other level of consciousness, for there is none external to Itself. Our individual consciousness, by habit, becomes absorbed by objects of attention, and fails to be aware of the Self, the Seer. One must restrain the outward pull of the senses and mental movements upon consciousness, and turn inwards. Be aware of the Self, the fundamental Presence permeating everything.

Practice: Practice being conscious of what is conscious.

21. *citta-antara-dṛśye buddhi-buddher-atiprasaṅgaḥ smṛti-saṃkaraś-ca*

citta=mind; consciousness

antara = other

dṛśye = perception

buddhi = the intellect; the first *tattva* to arise from *prakṛti*, in *Sāṁkhya* philosophy; perception; discrimination; mind

buddheḥ = of the intellect, perception; discrimination; mind

atiprasaṅgaḥ = excessive attachment; impertinence; here: infinite regression

smṛti=memory

saṅkara = confusion

ca = and

If the perception of one consciousness by another [consciousness] be postulated, we would have to assume an infinite regression of them and the result would be confusion of memory.

Patañjali rejects the suggestion that within an individual there could be an endless series of individualized consciousness, each aware of the other, because it would cause memory to stop functioning. There is only one Consciousness, within each individual; it becomes distorted by various movements. But when these mental distortions become silent, a higher universal Consciousness is awakened, and the feeling of possessing an individual body or personality dies.

Practice: Contemplate the existence of one Universal Consciousness permeating all forms.

22. *citer-apratisaṃkramāyā tad-ākāra-āpattau svabuddhi-saṃvedanam*

citeḥ = of transcendental consciousness; higher awareness

apratisaṃkramāyāḥ = because of or due to the unchanging, non-dissolution

tad = that

ākāra = form, figure, shape, appearance

āpattau = in, at concerning the happening, occurrence, arising; entering into a state of condition; here: assumes

svabuddhi = own intellect

saṃvedanam = perception

When the unchanging transcendental consciousness assumes the form of that [consciousness], perception of one's own intellect [becomes possible].

While the higher universal consciousness itself does not change, because of ignorance, it assumes the forms of the lower consciousness (see verse I.4). The consciousness of our own intellect, and mind, would not be possible without the closeness of the Self; for it illuminates the latter. But this false identification *(sārūpyam)* between the Self and individuated consciousness is only apparent. When the movements arising within consciousness subside, "Then the Seer (Self) abides in his own true form" (*tadā draṣṭuḥ sva-rūpe' vasthānam*, verse I.3).

Practice: Cultivate a mindset that lets go of all mental disturbances. Rest in the space between them. Be the Self.

23. *draṣṭṛ-dṛśya-uparaktaṃ cittaṃ sarva-artham*

draṣṭṛ = the Seer

dṛiśya = the seen

uparaktam = colored; tinted, dyed

cittaṃ = consciousness; mind

sarva = all

artham = meaning, purpose; aim; object

All objects of the mind are colored by the Seer and the Seen.

Earlier in verse IV.17, Patañjali indicated that an object (*vastu)* can be recognized by one's consciousness if it is colored (*uparāga)* by that object (that is, if there is a memory of it already). Here he states a second necessary condition for perception to occur: the individualized consciousness must be "colored" (*uparaktaḥ)* or "illumined" by the Self (or Seer). This second condition exists so long as one is alive and in one of the four states of consciousness: physical, dream (*svapna),* dreamless and the transcendental (*turya*). Individualized consciousness, however, because of ignorance or confusion over its true identity, regards the eternal unchanging Self as an object, and misses its true identity.

Practice: Remember the Self always.

24. *tad-asaṃkhyeya-vāsanābhiś-citram api para-arthaṃ saṃhatya-kāritvāt*

tad = that

asaṃkhyeya = countless; innumerable; multitude

vāsanābhiḥ = with or by subconscious impressions; habit patterns

citram = variegated, spotted, speckled; various

api = also

para-arthaṃ = the highest goal; the supreme; the interest of another; something else; an object meant for another's use

saṃhatya = together, simultaneously, all at a time

kāritvāt = because of or due to action or activity; effected

That [consciousness] though filled with countless subconscious impressions, exists for the sake of another [the Self] because it can act only in association with it.

The individual consciousness has as its purpose the realization of the Self. While it is filled with countless subconscious impressions, through the process of yogic purification, ultimately one goes beyond them to Self-realization. The mind's games may seem to serve lesser purposes. Once we discover this higher purpose, we begin to leave behind involvement in the mind's games, and we begin to play the game of consciousness. In this game, whenever we are aware, we "win": we experience joy. Whenever we forget to be aware, we lose: we suffer.

Practice: Play the game of Consciousness: practice joyful awareness at all times, in all situations, whether they be painful or pleasurable; practice the technique of continual bliss (*nityānanda kriyā)* as taught in *Babaji's Kriya Yoga* level II initiation.

25. *viśeṣa-darśina ātma-bhāva-bhāvanā-vinivṛttiḥ*

viśeṣa = distinction; peculiar mark; special property

darśinaḥ = seeing, perceiving, viewing, observing, knowing, understanding

ātmabhāva = existence of the Self or soul; the Self proper, peculiar nature;

bhāvana = cultivation; forebearance; meditation; observing; investigating

vinivṛttiḥ = turn back, withdrawn; cessation, stopping removing; ceases forever

To one who sees the distinction between seeing and the Self, there ceases forever the cultivation [of the false self-sense].

During elevated states of consciousness, such as deep meditation, one may reach the limit of individualized consciousness: pure seeing. Thoughts have already been left behind. At this limit one ceases to cultivate individualized consciousness, and effortlessly cultivates Self consciousness. "One loses the habit of thinking," as Aurobindo complained half jokingly, and one remains fixed in the awareness that one is the pure subject, universal and eternal.

This goes beyond the stage where one may ask mentally and repeatedly, "Who am I?" While such a mental inquiry may ultimately prepare one for "pure seeing," it is usually only the long process of *Yoga,* which can ultimately prepare and refine the individuated consciousness. How *asaṁprajñāta samādhi* brings about the extinction of individuated consciousness is indicated in the commentary on IV.27.

The sages say that when you are in this state of union with the Divine, you spend it laughing at all the things of this existence! You see the Divine everywhere and in everything, and there are no differences. And through this realization, nothing has the power to make you fall back into your old way of seeing. Nothing exists but That Consciousness, Presence, Power, Love, forever.

Once, there was a wandering a monk (*sādhu)* known as Chela Swami, who would visit the small village of Kanadukatan, in the Chettinad region of Tamil Nadu. He wore no clothes, and appeared to be mad. He came and went like the wind. He was always smiling. Naughty children would sometimes throw stones at him. He smiled. At other times they would treat him with kindness, and massage his feet. He would smile. Sometimes children would give him a banana. He would smile. Then they would snatch the banana away. Still he smiled. Why do you think he was always smiling?

Practice: Practice joyful awareness at all times.

26. *tadā viveka-nimnaṃ kaivalya-prāgbhāraṃ cittaṃ*

tadā = then, indeed

viveka = discernment;

nimnan = inclined towards;

kaivalya = aloneness; absolute freedom [see verse II.24]

prāgbhāram = gravitating toward; propensity, inclination;

citta = consciousness; mind

Then consciousness gravitates towards absolute freedom and is inclined towards discernment.

When only the thinnest veil of ignorance (*avidyā*), or confusion (*saṁkara*), between the Self and the non-Self remains, discernment (*viveka*) between these two continues automatically and one moves inexorably towards the highest form of *samādhi*. In II.25, this final state is defined as the absolute freedom from the seen (*dṛśeḥ kaivalyam*). There remains pure subjectivity of the root consciousness. Thoughts and sensations may continue, but there is no more feeling of being their owner or originator. Whatever action is performed, there is no more a sense of being the doer. One is only the Seer.

Kaivalyam as "aloneness" means neither seclusion, nor renunciation as such, but absolute freedom from the causes of affliction. Aloneness means being open to the Divine within always and allowing the Divine to work through oneself while being free from any personal preference. Aloneness means you are "All One," for no one else exists.

Practice: Be "alone" in a crowd. Let nothing affect your peace and equanimity, regardless of what is happening around you.

27. *tac-chidreṣu pratyaya-antarāṇi saṃskārebhyaḥ*

tat = this; that

chidreṣu = torn asunder, containing holes, pierced, defect, fault, between

pratyaya = intention; thought, notion, cognition

antarāṇi = others

saṃskāra = subconscious impressions

In between, other thoughts [may arise] due to subconscious impressions.

This highest state of absolute freedom of the Seer (*dṛśeḥ kaivalyam*) or non-distinguished cognitive absorption (*asaṁprajñāta samādhi*) will generally be manifested for only short periods in the beginning. Subconscious impressions (*saṁskāras)* will continue to disturb the emerging higher consciousness. Gradually, the *yogin* remembers to let go of all externalizing impressions, except for that of detachment (*vairāgya)* itself. Finally the movement inward outweighs the externalizing movement of consciousness until clear Self-consciousness remains.

Practice: Practice being the witness, seeing all distraction (*vikṣepa*) as waves on the surface of your ocean of Being. Be the ocean, not the waves.

28. *hānam-eṣāṃ kleśavad-uktam*

hānam = abandoned, forsaken, extinguished; removed

eṣām = of those

kleśavat = like affliction

uktam = spoken

They can be removed like the afflictions [as explained previously].

Here Patañjali reminds us how to remove these distracting thoughts by referring back to verses II.1, 2, 10, 11 and 26, wherein he explains the afflictions (*kleśas)* and how to remove to them.

Practice: See all disturbances as an opportunity to cultivate equanimity (*upekṣa)* and inner stillness. Gradually the time will lessen between when you feel disturbed and when you return to your center.

29. *prasaṃkhyāne' py-akusīdasya sarvathā viveka-khyāter-dharma-meghaḥ samādhiḥ*

prasaṃkhyāne = in the attainment; enumeration, reflection meditation
api = even

akusīdasya = of non-interest in rewards or gain

sarvathā = constant; at all times, always

viveka = discriminative

khyāteḥ = of discernment [see verse II.26 and II.28]

dharma = essential character; nature, character

megha = cloud

samādhiḥ = cognitive absorption

Disinterested in rewards and remaining in discriminative discernment at all times, there follows the state of cognitive absorption known as the cloud of *dharma*.

The term "*dharma* cloud" or "cloud of *dharma*" is not described any further, but given the characteristics of its preparation, it must necessarily occur just before the attainment of non-distinguished cognitive absorption (*asaṁprajñātaḥ samādhi*), ultra-cognitive (seedless or *nirbija*) absorption. This may be similar to *dharmakaya* or "body of truth" in Buddhism, the experience of vacuity of emptiness. Discriminative discernment (*viveka-khyāteḥ*) was described in II.26 and II.28, as the means of separating the Self from the world. It essentially consists of first stepping back from all the movements occurring within consciousness and later stepping back from individual consciousness into the "root consciousness of the Self."

In such a state, the person becomes freed from the pull of "the pairs of opposites" in dualistic thinking (right and wrong, beautiful and ugly, etc.) and *dharmic* principles of righteous conduct or duty become superfluous. With no sense of "I" or "mine," there is no corresponding sense of duty. One desires nothing. One has no need to do anything. While the body still may exist, due to force of past *karma*, the *yogin* is not affected by it. His bodily actions and also actions in the surface mind continue until this *karma* is exhausted.

Practice: As consciousness expands, and the heart opens, do not allow them to be dispersed into mental movements, such as memories, fantasies, sensual indulgences. Turn them towards the Divine, and in so doing; maintain purity, contentment and discernment.

30. *tataḥ kleśa-karma-nivṛttiḥ*

tatas = from that

kleśa = afflictions

karma = action

nivṛtti = cessation

From that, there is the cessation of afflictions and action.

In the *dharma* cloud (*dharma-meghaḥ) samādhi,* the background comes to the foreground and what is in the foreground during ordinary physical consciousness recedes to the background. One never again loses sight of the absolute Reality. One is no longer moved by afflictions. (see verse I.24). One ceases to be affected by past actions or to create new *karma.* One's consciousness has arisen to a higher, transcendental state. There is no longer the sense of "I-am-the-doer." One awakens from the dream.

However, this does not preclude the performance of action nor remaining in the world, as some have argued, based upon a *Sāṁkhya* based opposition of Self-realization to world involvement.**(15)** As shown earlier, the *Tamil Yoga Siddhas* sought not to leave the world, but to transform their own involvement in it, allowing the descent of a higher consciousness into all the levels of their being, including the physical. However, if one acts, it is not with the sense of being the doer, much less out of any ego bound motivation. One may be in the world, but not of it. Why remain in the world? The *Siddhas* indicated repeatedly that if they remain, it is only to serve the divine transformation of others who are ripening. This is not very different from *bodhisattva* to either refrain from attaining supreme enlightenment until all beings can do so with him or her; or, achieving enlightenment solely for the benefit of all sentient beings; or once achieving enlightenment, remaining in the world for as long as there is suffering. *Santideva* has said in his *Bodhi sattva caryavartara*" that so long as there is suffering in the world, so too will I remain".**(16)**

Practice: Practice silence regularly. Speak only when it is necessary and edifying for others, after reflection. Avoid the trap of pride of attainment, by cultivating silence. Do not try to communicate or conceptualize the Realization that comes; such efforts will only bring down the consciousness.

31. *tadāsarva-āvaraṇa-mala-apetasya jñānasya-ānantyāj-jñeyam-alpam*

tadā = then

sarva = all

āvaraṇa = covering

mala = impurity, dirt, filth, dust

apetasya = of the departed; removal

jñānaysa = of the wisdom

ānantyāt = because of the infinite, the eternal

jñeyam = to be known

alpam = little; small

Then all the coverings and impurities of wisdom are removed. Because of the infinity of this wisdom, what remains to be known is almost nothing.

Normally our consciousness is absorbed or dispersed by objects of attention due to the presence of imperfections, including desire (*rāgāḥ*), memory (*smṛtiḥ*), ego (*asmitā*) and aversion (*dveṣaḥ*). But when these are removed our consciousness can reflect the "Absolute Reality" without judgment or division. Letting go of the confusion of the mind, the Self finds identity with the underlying reality of all. All phenomena becomes transparent in an infinite, eternal field of

Being. This is wisdom, and unlike knowledge, it is non-dual, is limitless, and is apprehended intuitively, by becoming one with its object.

Practice: Reflect upon the difference between knowing and being.

32. *tataḥ kṛta-arthānāṃ pariṇāma-krama-samāptir-guṇānām*

tatas = then; from that

kṛta = done; here: achieved or fulfilled

arthānām = of purposes

pariṇāma = transformation

krama = sequence; succession

samāptiḥ = termination; conclusion, accomplishment

guṇānām = of the qualities or modes of nature

Then the gunas terminate their sequence of transformations because they have fulfilled their purpose.

Having transcended the states of waking, dreaming and deep sleep, the adept abides in the fourth state (*turīya*), and therefore ceases to be involved in, or subject to, the qualities of nature (*guṇas*).

Sattvic is *Guṇa* in the Waking state
Rajas in Dream state
Tamas in Deep Sleep state
Nirguṇa, that other three *Guṇas* destroys
Is attribute of *Turīya* State Pure. (TM 2296)

And

When that State is attained
Where the Self becomes Śiva
The *Malas* (stains), the *Pasas* (*Tam.* fetters) diverse
Guṇas and experiences

That arose for the estranged *Jīva*
Will all, all fade.
Even as does the beams of the moon
In the presence of the rising sun. (TM2314)

The *guṇa's* purpose has been to provide the setting and functions wherein the individual soul (*jīva*) could go beyond its ignorance, and return to union with the Supreme Lord. Now they fade into the background, in the light of Self-realization.

Practice: Reflect on the advice of the *Yoga* of qualified non-dualism (*yoga-vāśiṣṭha*): "Leave untouched whatever is tangible or can be obtained through your own agency; remain unaffected and independent of anything in the world, and rely on your consciousness of infinity. Think of yourself as sleeping when your are awake; think of yourself as all, and as one with the supreme Spirit."**(17)**

33. *kṣaṇa-pratiyogī pariṇāma-apara-anta-nirgrāhyaḥ kramaḥ*

kṣaṇa = moment

pratiyogī = correlate; counterpart

pariṇāma = transformation

aparānta = end

nirgrāhyaḥ = terminated; cease; to be suppressed

kramaḥ = sequence; succession

Succession and [its] counterpart, the moment, cease with the end of transformation.

Having reached the highest state of transcendental consciousness, one recognizes the eternal changeless One behind the apparent changes. "Be Still and know that I am God" is another way of referring to what Patañjali says in this verse. In the stillness, in the silence, the end of changes is realized. The wave merges back into the ocean of being. The mind has divided our experience of reality into finite pieces: moments, experiences, thoughts, sensations. Having gone beyond the mind, into *samādhi,* one now realizes union of everything. When we awaken from the dream of life, it resembles the realization that occurs when we come to the end of a movie that we have been engrossed in. We see our whole life in reverse like a series of images on the videotape being rewound.

Practice: Contemplate the paradox, which this implies: after finishing the journey, one returns to where one began, and realizes that what one was seeking was there all the time.

34. *puruṣa-artha-śūnyānāṃ guṇānāṃ pratiprasavaḥ kaivalyaṃ svarūpa-pratiṣṭhā vā citi-śaktir-iti*

puruṣārtha = the goal of man; the purpose of the self

śūnyānāṁ = of being empty

guṇānāṁ = of the qualities or constituent forces of nature.

pratiprasavaḥ = reabsorb; returning to the origin or source

kaivalyam = aloneness; absolute freedom, independence

svarūpa = own nature or form in and of itself; see verse I.3

pratiṣṭhā = establishment; steadfastness; perseverance settles in

vā = or

citiśakti = power of pure consciousness or higher awareness

iti = thus

Thus the supreme state of Absolute freedom manifests while the qualities reabsorb themselves into Nature, having no more purpose to serve the Self. Or [from another angle], the power of

pure consciousness settles in its own pure Nature.

In this final verse, Patañjali characterizes the supreme, absolute state of realization as absolute freedom (*kaivalyam),* and tells us that it involves the union of Consciousness (*puruṣa*) with Nature (*prakṛti*). This verse echoes that of I.3 "Then the Seer abides in his true form" (*tadā draṣṭuḥ sva-rūpe' vasthānam).* While these are terms which are found throughout *Sāṁkhya Kārikās* and the *Vedāntas,* their use here can be better understood within the context of earlier verses in particular, (see I.16, 24, III.35, 49, 55, IV.18) and the *Tamil Yoga Siddha* philosophy in general.

In the terms used by the *Tamil Yoga Siddhas,* this is the union of *Ś*iva (Supreme consciousness) with *śakti (*power). As a result of this union within the *yogin,* a radical transformation takes place at all levels. The lower Nature, previously motivated only by the constituent forces of Nature (*guṇas),* is replaced by a higher form of Nature (*svarūpa*): one's own true form or Nature. Initiates of *Babaji's Kriya Yoga* will recognize this as the *svarūpa samādhi* or golden *samādhi* referred to throughout the Tamil *Yoga Siddha* literature. In it, even the cells of the physical body surrender their limited modes and agendas to that of a *samādhi-*based consciousness, and glow with golden light. All of the *Siddhas* in the 18 Tamil *Yoga Siddha* tradition referred to this *svarūpa samādhi* and described how their bodies glowed so brightly with a golden luster. So did the 19th century *Siddha Ramalinga Swami,* who referred to it as the "body of Supreme Grace Light."**(18)** So did Sri Aurobindo, who referred to it as the "descent of the supramental."**(19)** The laws of a lower nature with the action of the constituent forces of nature (*guṇas*) are replaced by that of a higher Nature. All of them spoke from their own personal experience at this final stage of supreme transformation.

> What is the sign of *svarūpa mukti* [the liberation of form in and of itself]?
> The physical body glows with the
> Fire of immortality. - Roma Rishi

Tirumūlar refers to *svarūpa* as "Self-illuminating manifestness" in dozens of verses:

> *Jīva* having become *Śiva*
> And the triple *Malas* extinguished,

Ascending into Triple Spaces
In Desire and Not-desire ceased
Pass into the body state of
Satya-Jñāna-ānanda Bliss;
There in that furthest *Turīya* of *Jīva*
The Self-illuminating Manifestness (*svarūpa*) is. (TM 2834)

And The Holy Master, *Parama Guru* (supreme *guru*)
As *Para* constant pervades interminably all
In that immanent state
Extends His Self-Illuminating Manifestness (*svarūpa*),
When *Jīva* the Final *Turīya* State attains. (TM 2835)

In this "Final Turīya State," the individual soul (*jīva),* becomes undifferentiated in the Supreme Being, and attains the subtle *Śiva* state of Luminous Self-Manifestness. Whether the *yogin* in this state continues to manifest a body in this world, or not, is beside the point; one is no longer subject to the ordinary laws and constituent forces of Nature. If one leaves this world, it will not be because one is forced to do so because of decay and death. As Babaji has said "Death is a joke to me, as I am the Death of Death."**(20)**

The one is always alone:

Transcend *Kalas* Five,
In the Waking State (of *Turīya*) appear;
Reach the lonely State of Higher *Kevala*
And there solitary be;
Bereft of sentience,
Ardent enter the (*Turīya) atita* State:
Then shall you the very *Tat-Para* be. (TM 2450)

"Blessed sister", Babaji said, "I am intending to shed my form and plunge into the Infinite Current."

"I have already glimpsed your plan, beloved master. I wanted to discuss it with you tonight. Why should you leave your body?" The glorious woman looked at him beseechingly. "What is the difference if I wear a visible or invisible wave on the ocean of my Spirit?" Mataji replied with a quaint flash of wit. "Deathless guru, if it makes no difference, then please do not ever relinquish your form."

"Be it so," Babaji said solemnly. "I will never leave my physical body. It will always remain visible to at least a small number of people on this earth. The Lord has spoken His own wish through your lips... Fear not, Ram Gopal" he said, "you are blessed to be a witness at the scene of this immortal promise."... Lahiri Mahasaya later explained to me many metaphysical points concerning the hidden divine plan for this earth, Gopal concluded. "Babaji has been chosen by God to remain in his body for the duration of this particular world cycle. Ages shall come and go - still the deathless master beholding the drama of the centuries, shall be present on this stage terrestrial."**(21)**

Practice: Imagine the presence of a living Divine Person, like Babaji, free of the limitations of the qualities or constituent forces of nature, and the limited functioning of the ordinary mind and body. Learn and practice *vijñāna Babaji darśana kriyā* as revealed in the *Babaji's Kriya Yoga* level III initiation.

AUM TAT SAT

OṂ KRIYĀ BABAJI NĀMA AUM

Patañjali's Kriya Yoga Sūtras Continuous Translation of the 195 Sūtras

Chapter 1: SAMĀDHI-PĀDA
Cognitive Absorption

1. Now [begins] the exposition of Yoga.
2. Yoga is the cessation [of identifying with] the fluctuations [arising within] consciousness.
3. Then the Seer abides in his own true form.
4. Otherwise, there is an identification [by the individuated self] with the fluctuations [of consciousness].
5. The fluctuations [of consciousness] are five-fold, being afflicted and unafflicted.
6. These five are: the means of acquiring true knowledge, misconception, conceptualization, sleep and memory.
7. The means of obtaining true knowledge are: perception via the five senses, inference and the study of sacred works.
8. Misconception is false knowledge not based upon it's true form.
9. Conceptualization is the result of knowledge [acquired from] verbal communication having no real abiding substance.
10. The fluctuation of sleep is based on a belief in non-existence.
11. Memory is not letting an object experienced be carried away [from ones consciousness].
12. By constant practice and with detachment [arises] the cessation [of identifying with the fluctuations of consciousness].
13. In this context, the effort to abide in [the cessation of identification with the fluctuations of consciousness] is a constant practice.
14. However, this [practice only becomes] firmly established when properly and consistently attended to over a long [period of] time.
15. Detachment is the emblem of the mastery of one who sees and hears an object without craving.
16. That freedom from the constituent forces [of nature] [which arises] due to an individual's [Self]-realization is supreme.
17. Distinguished [*saṁprajñāta*] cognitive absorption is accompanied by observation, reflecting, rejoicing and awareness of the Self.

18. Preceded by constant practice with the contemplation of detachment, [there is the] other [state of cognitive absorption, i.e. a non-distinguished cognitive absorption which possesses] residual subconscious impressions.
19. Of those [*yogin's*] who [being] disincarnate are absorbed into nature [there is] the intention of becoming.
20. For other [*yogins*], [the accomplishment of non-distinguished cognitive absorption] is preceded by intense devotion, courage, mindfulness, cognitive absorption and true insight.
21. [For those practitioners who are] utterly resolute [in their practice, the accomplishment of cognitive absorption] is imminent.
22. Thus, the characteristic difference [as to how quickly spiritual union] is reached depends [on whether the *yogin's* practice] is weak, moderate or intense.
23. Or, because of [one's] surrender to the Lord [one successfully achieves absorption].
24. *Ishvara* is the special Self, untouched by any afflictions, actions, fruits of actions or by any inner impressions of desires.
25. There [in the Supreme] the seed of the [manifestation of complete] omniscience is unsurpassed.
26. Unconditioned by time, he is the teacher of even the most ancient teachers.
27. The word expressive [of *īśvara*] is the mystic sound *OM* [*AUM*].
28. Therefore, one should] repeat [this sacred syllable *Oṁ*] while reflecting on its meaning with devotion.
29. [From this practice] comes the attainment of the "inner Self awareness" and the disappearance of [all] obstacles.
30. Disease, dullness, doubt, carelessness, laziness, sense indulgence, false perception, failure to reach firm ground and instability - these distractions of consciousness are obstacles.
31. The accompaniments of [these] distractions are trembling in the body, unsteady inhalation, (of the breath) depression and anxiety.
32. The practice of concentration on a single subject is the best way to prevent [the obstacles and their accompaniments].
33. By cultivating attitudes of friendship towards the happy, compassion for the unhappy, delight in the virtuous and equanimity towards the non-virtuous the concsiousness retains its undisturbed calmness.
34. Or [that undisturbed calmness of consciousness is achieved] by the [careful] exhalation and the retention of the breath.
35. Or the holding of the mind steady is brought about by cognitive [focus with in] the field [of the senses].

36. Or [by concentrating on the] ever blissful supreme light within [one leaves behind all suffering and one experiences lucidity].
37. Or [that undisturbed calmness of mind is achieved when] consciousness [is directed towards the minds of those great souls] who have conquered attachment.
38. Or [that undisturbed calmness of mind] is supported by the knowledge that arises in dreams and sleep.
39. Or from the subject of meditation [choosing anything] as desired.
40. [Gradually one's] mastery [of concentration] extends from the most minute [primal atom] to the greatest magnitude.
41. Just as a pure crystal assumes the colors [or shapes] of objects standing nearby, so cognitive absorption [occurs] when the fluctuations [of consciousness], having dwindled [by various means], knower, known and their relationship becomes indistinguishable.
42. The cognitive absorption wherein subject-object identification is mixed with spontaneous words, objects and knowledge about material objects, is known as "*savitarkā samadhi*": *Samadhi* with reflection.
43. The cognitive absorption wherein subject-object identification is well purified of impressions, and one has become, as it were, empty, in one's own form only, shining without reflection is "*nirvitarkā samādhi.*"
44. Similarly explained are the [states of cognitive absorption wherein the subject-object identification] is mixed with words and reflections about subtle objects, "*savicara*" [*samadhi*] and without words and reflections, "*nirvicara*" [*samadhi*].
45. The subtle nature of objects terminate in the unmanifest.
46. These very cognitive absorptions possess seed (s).
47. In the pristine state of *nirvicāra samādhi* [absorption without words and reflection] the supreme Self [shines] in undisturbed calmness.
48. In that [*nirvicāra samādhi*] [state of absorption without words and reflection] awareness is truth bearing.
49. This special truth has a distinct purpose apart from knowledge, inference, or scriptural study.
50. The subconscious impressions produced from that [truth bearing awareness] will impede [the arising of any] other subconscious impressions.
51. With the cessation [of identifying with] even this last impression, ["I am,"] all [others] having been restrained, there results the seedless "*nirbija*" cognitive *samadhi.*

Chapter 2: SADHANA-PĀDA
Discipline

1. Intense practice, self-study and devotion to the Lord constitute *kriyā yoga*.
2. [They are used] for the purpose of weakening [any] affliction [and] cultivating cognitive absorption.
3. Ignorance, egoism, attachment, aversion and clinging to life are the five afflictions.
4. Ignorance is the field [from which other] afflictions [arise] and can be dormant, weak, intercepted or active.
5. Ignorance is seeing the impermanent as permanent, the impure as pure, the painful as pleasurable and the non-Self as the Self.
6. Egoism is the identification, as it were, of the powers of the Seer [Purusha] with that of the instrument of seeing [body-mind].
7. Attachment is the clinging to pleasure.
8. Aversion is clinging to suffering.
9. Clinging to life [which] is self-sustaining, arises even in the wise.
10. These [afflictions in their] subtle [form], are destroyed by tracing [their] cause[s] back to [their] origin.
11. [In the active state], these fluctuations [arising within consciousness] are destroyed by meditation.
12. The reservoir of *karmas* rooted in the afflictions, is experienced in seen [present] and unseen [future] existence.
13. So long as the root exists, [its] fruits also exist; [namely] birth, and [it's] experiences.
14. Because of virtuous and non-virtuous *karma*, there are [corresponding] pleasurable and painful consequences.
15. Because of the conflict between the fluctuations [of consciousness] and the constituent forces of nature, and with the suffering [that arises from] the subconscious impressions, anxiety and change, for the discriminating person, indeed all is sorrowful.
16. [That which is] to be eliminated is future sorrow.
17. The cause [of suffering] to be eliminated is the union of the Seer and the Seen.
18. The Seen is of the quality of brightness, activity and inertia; and consists of the elements and sense organs whose purpose is [to provide both] experience and liberation [to the Self].
19. The divisions of the primary constituent forces of nature are specific, non-specific, defined and undefinable.

20. [Being] pure, the Seer, through the power of merely seeing [directly] perceives thoughts.
21. The Seen [exists] only for the sake of the Self.
22. For one who has attained the goal [of liberation, the Seen] disappears; [yet, the Seen] is not destroyed because of its common universality.
23. The union of Owner [*puruṣa*] and owned [*prakṛti*] causes the recognition of the essence and power of them both.
24. The cause of this union is ignorance.
25. Without this ignorance [*avidyā*], no such union [*saṁyoga*] occurs. This is the absolute freedom [*kaivalyam*] from the Seen [*dṛśeḥ*].
26. Uninterrupted discriminative discernment is the method for its removal.
27. One's wisdom in the final stage is sevenfold.
28. By the practice of the limbs of Yoga, the impurities dwindle away and there dawns the light of wisdom leading to discriminative discernment.
29. The eight limbs of Yoga are: *yama*/restraint, *niyama*/observance, *asana*/posture, *pranayama*/breath control, *pratyahara*/sense withdrawal, *dharana*/concentration, *dhyana*/meditation, and *samadhi*/cognitive absorption.
30. The restraints are non-violence, truthfulness, non-stealing, chastity and greedlessness.
31. This Great Vow is universal, not limited by class, place, time or circumstances.
32. Observances [*niyamas*] consist of purity, contentment, accepting but not causing pain, self-study and surrender to the Lord.
33. [When] bound by negative thoughts, [their] opposite [i.e. positive] ones should be cultivated. [This is] *pratipakṣa bhāvanam.*
34. When negative thoughts or acts such as violence, etc. are caused to be done or even approved of, whether incited by greed, anger or infatuation, whether indulged in with mild, moderate or extreme intensity, they are based on ignorance and bring certain pain. [Hence] Opposite thoughts should be cultivated.
35. In the presence of one firmly established in non-violence, all hostilities cease.
36. To one established in truthfulness, actions and their results depend upon [him].
37. Wealth comes to all established in non-stealing.

38. By one established in chastity, vigor is gained.
39. When greedlessness is established, illuminated knowledge of the how and why of one's birth comes.
40. By purification arises disgust for one's own body and no contact with other [bodies].
41. Moreover one gains purity of being, joy in the mind, one-pointedness, mastery over the senses and fitness for Self-realization.
42. By contentment, supreme joy is gained.
43. By austerity, impurities of the body and senses are destroyed and perfection is gained.
44. By self-study [comes] communion with one's chosen deity.
45. Because of [one's] surrender to the Lord, cognitive absorption is attained.
46. *Āsana* is a steady, comfortable posture.
47. From the relaxation of tension and endless unity [*samadhi* is established].
48. Thereafter one is invulnerable to the dualities.
49. With regard to [these postures] breath control is the control of the motions of inhalation and exhalation.
50. Breath control is external, internal or stationary. It is perceived according to time, space and number and [becomes long and subtle].
51. There is a fourth during withdrawal [between] internal and external conditions [of breathing].
52. As a result, the veil over [the inner] Light is destroyed.
53. And the mind becomes fit for concentration.
54. When the senses disunite themselves from their own objects and imitate, as it were, their own form of consciousness, this is sense withdrawal.
55. Then [you should have] supreme mastery over the senses.

Chapter 3: VIBHŪTI-PĀDA
Extraordinary Powers

1. Concentration is the binding of consciousness to one place, object or idea.
2. In this context, meditation is the experience of having the mind fixed on one object only.

3. Cognitive absorption [*samādhiḥ*] is that meditation [when] the whole object [i.e. consciousness] shines forth, as if devoid of its own form.
4. The practice of these three [*dhāraṇā, dhyāna and samādhi*] together upon one object is communion [*saṁyama*].
5. Due to the mastery [of communion] the light of insight arises.
6. It's progression is in stages.
7. These three [*dhāraṇā, dhyāna and samādhi*] are more internal than the preceding five limbs.
8. These three are indeed the outer limbs of the seedless cognitive absorption [*samādhi*].
9. When the restless [movements] arising within consciousness are overpowered and subside [by the action] of restraint, there follows, in that moment, the development of the subconscious impression of restraint.
10. The calm flow of cleansing transformation develops through subconscious impressions.
11. When there is a decline in objectification and [there is an] appearance of one-pointedness, [there arises] the development of the cognitive absorption [*samādhi*] of the mind.
12. Hence, when the intentions that direct the repeated arising and subsiding [of thoughts] become similar, there is a transformation [into a] one-pointedness of consciousness.
13. By this, concerning the sense organs and the elements, the transformation of the quality, character and condition [of the mind] have been fully detailed.
14. It is [that which is] subject to the particular laws of nature [i.e. *prakṛti*] [whose] nature is undisturbed, manifested, and undetermined.
15. The differentiation in the sequences [of these different phases] is the cause in the differences in [stages of] evolution.
16. From communion in the three-fold [stage of] evolution [arises] knowledge of the past and future.
17. Because of the superimposition of words, purposes and intentions with one another, [there arises] confusion; [however], through communion [focused on distinguishing them], knowledge of all things [is attained].
18. Knowledge of previous births [arises] because of the intuitive perception of subconscious impressions.

19. [Similarly, because of the intuitive perception of another's] intention [one is capable of] knowing the thoughts of another.
20. But [knowing another's thoughts] is without [an actual] basis because there is no object in the elements.
21. Through communion on the form of the body, upon suspension of the capacity to be perceived, upon the disruption of light [traveling from that body] invisibility to the eye [follows].
22. *Karma* is either latent or manifest. From communion on this or on the signs of approaching death, [arises] the knowledge of death.
23. [By communion] on friendliness and other such qualities, the power [to transmit them is attained].
24. [By communion] on the powers of elephants and other [such animals], their strength [is obtained].
25. By communion with the illuminated inner senses, the knowledge of the subtle, concealed and remote is obtained.
26. From communion on the sun, knowledge of the world and cosmic regions is obtained.
27. [By communion] on the moon [comes] knowledge [of the] stars' arrangements.
28. [By communion] on the pole star comes knowledge [of the] stars' movements.
29. [By communion] on the wheel of the navel, knowledge of the body's constitution is obtained.
30. [By communion] on the throat cavity, cessation of hunger and thirst is achieved.
31. [By communion] on the tortoise channel, motionlessness [is achieved].
32. [By communion] on the light [at the crown of] the head, a vision of perfected ones is obtained.
33. Or, all [the powers come by themselves through] a flash of illumination.
34. [By communion] at the heart, knowledge [of the nature of] consciousness [is obtained].
35. [When there is] an ulterior motive, the resultant experience is [that there is] no distinction [between] the awareness of manifest being in nature and the Self; [when one practices] communion for its own sake, [one obtains] self-knowledge.
36. Thus, spontaneous intuitive flashes [based in] hearing, touching, seeing, tasting, and smelling are produced.

37. These attainments are obstacles to cognitive absorption but are accomplishments in the waking state.
38. Due to the relaxation of the cause of bondage and the knowledge of manifestation, entering into another body of consciousness [can take place].
39. By mastery over the vital force in the upper part of the body [the adept gains the power of] imperviousness to water, mud and thorns [as well as the power of] levitation.
40. By mastery of the vital force in the abdominal region [here is] radiance.
41. [By communion] on the relationship between the ear and ether, there is clairaudience.
42. [By communion] on the relationship between the body and space, and [by being in a state of] cognitive absorption [focused upon] light [objects, such as] cotton, [the power to travel across] space [is gained].
43. During this great out of body experience, the fluctuations arising within consciousness are inconceivable, as they are perceived to be external to this body, and from this, comes the dwindling of the veil over the light of the Self.
44. By communion with the objects [of nature] at their coarse and subtle levels and on their essence, correlations and purpose, mastery over the five elements is gained.
45. Then [comes] the manifestation of powers such as bodily perfection and invulnerability of its functions.
46. Beauty, grace, strength and extraordinary endurability [constitute] perfection of the body.
47. By communion with the [power of] perception and on one's essential nature, as well as ego, their correlation and purpose, one gains mastery over the sense organs.
48. From this comes quickness of the mind, superphysical sensory capability, and mastery over the primary cause.
49. By seeing the distinction between the Self and being, [the adept] gains supremacy over all states [of existence] and omniscience.
50. Through detachment even towards [the *siddhis* of omniscience and omnipotence with] the destruction of the seed of this obstacle, there arises absolute freedom.
51. [Even] at the invitation of celestial beings [the adept should] not indulge any attachment or pride [because] undesired and renewed lower tendencies [may develop].

52. There is knowledge born from the arising of discrimination due to communion on the succession of instantaneous moments of time.
53. Hence there is the ascertainment of two similar [things], [owing to the fact that] they are not being limited by differences of origination, markings and place.
54. And, it is said that, the knowledge born of discrimination is liberating, non-sequential and [inclusive] of all conditions and all times.
55. In the sameness of purity between beingness and the Self, there is absolute freedom.

Chapter 4: KAIVALYA-PĀDA
Absolute Freedom

1. The powers are the results of birth, herbs, *mantras*, intense practice and cognitive absorption.
2. The transformation into another species [is due to] the vast possibilities inherent in Nature.
3. Incidental events do not [directly] cause natural evolution, but remove the obstacles as a farmer [removes the obstacles in a water course running to his field].
4. The individualized consciousness only [arises] from the limitation of egoism
5. [Although there is individualized consciousness] in different activities, the initiator is the one consciousness of the many other [individualized consciousnesses].
6. There [what arises] from meditation is without residue.
7. The *karma* of the *yogin* is neither white nor black; [but the *karma* of] others is threefold.
8. Hence, only those subconscious impressions for which there are favorable conditions for producing their fruits, will manifest.
9. As memory and residual subsconscious impressions are of one form, there is a link even [with] the separation of birth, place, time.
10. These [impressions] are beginningless, because desires are eternal.
11. The impressions being held together by cause, effect, basis and support, they disappear with the disappearance of these four.
12. The past and future exist in the real form of objects which manifest due to differences in the flow of forms [produced by

Nature].

13. These [forms] have manifest and subtle constituent forces of Nature.
14. From the oneness of transformation, there is the reality of an object.
15. Due to multiplicity of consciousness, the way of [perception] of even the same objects may vary.
16. Nor does an object's existence depend upon a single consciousness, for if it did, what would become of that object when that consciousness did not perceive it?
17. An object is known or unknown dependent on [upon] whether or not the consciousness gets colored by it.
18. The fluctuations of consciousness are always known, because of the changelessness of the Self, [who is] master.
19. That [fluctuations of consciousness] are not self-luminous because they are seen [objects].
20. Consequently, consciousness cannot perceive both [subject and object] simultaneously.
21. If the perception of one consciousness by another [consciousness] be postulated, we would have to assume an infinite regression of them and the result would be confusion of memory.
22. When the unchanging transcendental consciousness assumes the form of that [consciousness], perception of one's own intellect [becomes possible].
23. All objects of the mind are colored by the Seer and the Seen.
24. That [consciousness] though filled with countless subconscious impressions, exists for the sake of another [the Self] because it can act only in association with it.
25. To one who sees the distinction between seeing and the Self, there ceases forever the cultivation [of the false self-sense].
26. Then consciousness gravitates towards absolute freedom and is inclined towards discernment.
27. In between, other thoughts [may arise] due to subconscious impressions.
28. They can be removed like the afflictions [as explained previously].
29. Disinterested in rewards and remaining in discriminative discernment at all times, there follows the state of cognitive absorption known as the cloud of *dharma*.
30. From that, there is the cessation of afflictions and action.
31. Then all the coverings and impurities of wisdom are removed.

Because of the infinity of this wisdom, what remains to be known is almost nothing.

32. Then the gunas terminate their sequence of transformations because they have fulfilled their purpose.

33. Succession and [its] counterpart, the moment, cease with the end of transformation.

34. Thus the supreme state of Absolute freedom manifests while the qualities reabsorb themselves into Nature, having no more purpose to serve the Self. Or [from another angle], the power of pure consciousness settles in its own pure nature.

AUM TAT SAT

Notes to Introduction and Chapters

Introduction Part 1

1. Govindan, M. Editor, "Thirumandiram: A Classic of Yoga and Tantra," by Siddha Thirumoolar, 3rd edition, Kriya Yoga Publications, St. Etienne de Bolton, Quebec, Canada, 2003
2. Ganapathy, T. N. page 36, page 59 refers to 15 different lists of the 18 Siddhas
3. Feuerstein, Georg, "The Yoga-Sutra of Patanjali: A New Translation and Commentary," Inner Traditions, Rochester, Vermont, 1989
4. Satchitananda, Swami, "Integral Yoga: the Yoga Sutras of Patanjali," Integral Yoga Publications, Buckingham, Virginia, 1984
5. Aranya, Swami Hariharananda, "Yoga Philosophy of Patanjali," University of Calcutta Press, 48 Hazra Road, Calcutta, 700019
6. White, David Gordon, "The Alchemical Body: Siddha Traditions in Medieval India," University of Chicago Press, Chicago, 60637, 1996
7. Zvelebil, Kamil V. "The Poets of the Powers: Freedom, Magic, and Renewal," Integral Publishing, Lower Lake, California, 1993. Now solely distributed by Kriya Yoga Publications, St. Etienne de Bolton, Quebec, Canada.
8. Govindan, M. "Babaji and the 18 Siddha Kriya Yoga Tradition," 8th edition, Kriya Yoga Publications, St. Etienne de Bolton, Quebec, Canada, 2005

Introduction Part 2

1. Feuerstein, Georg, "The Sutras of Patanjali," A New Translation and Commentary," Inner Traditions, Rochester, Vermont, 1989 page 78.

2. Feuerstein, Georg, "Yoga Sutra: An Exercise in the Methodology of Textual Analysis," New Delhi, 1979. Available from the author at the Yoga Research and Education Center, P.O. box 1386, Lower Lake, California, USA, 95457
3. Feuerstein, Georg, "The Sutras of Patanjali," A New Translation and Commentary", Inner Traditions, Rochester, Vermont, 1989 page 59-60
4. Govindan, M. Editor, "Thirumandiram: A Classic of Yoga and Tantra" by Siddha Tirumular, 3rd edition, Babaji's Kriya Yoga and Publications, Eastman, Quebec, Canada J0E 1P0, 2003 verses 67 and 2790.

Chapter 1: SAMĀDHI-PĀDA

1. Aranya, Swami Hariharanananda, "Yoga Philosophy of Patanjali," page 41
2. T.N. Ganapathy, "The Philosophy of the Tamil Yoga Siddhas," page 30
3. K. Kailasapathay, "The writings of the Tamil Yoga Siddhas," page 313
4. L. Rose, "Your Mind: The Owner's Manual," published by Kriya Yoga Publications
5. T. N. Ganapathy, "The Philosophy of the Tamil Yoga Siddhas," page 71
6. G. Feuerstein, "The Yoga Sutra of Patanjali," page 76

Chapter 2: SĀDHANA-PĀDA

1. Feuerstein, G. Yoga Sutras, page 60
2. Ibid., page 60
3. Ibid., page 76
4. Ibid., page 78
5. Ibid., page 79
6. Feuerstein, G. "Holy Madness"
7. Rose, L. "Your Mind: the Owner's anual"
8. Aurobindo, Sri, "Letters on Yoga," page 1424-1589
9. Feuerstein, G. "Yoga Sutras", page 89

Chapter 3: VIBHŪTI-PĀDA

1. Aurobindo, Sri. "Sri Aurobindo on Himself, Reminiscences and Observations," page 356
2. The Mother, "The Mother's Agenda," 1962, Vol.3, page 201-204
3. Aranya, Swami Haranananda, page 299-302
4. Aranya, Swami Haranananda, page 304-305
5. The Mother, "The Mother's Agenda," 1962, Vol. 3, May 29, page 175
6. Aurobindo, Sri. "Letters on Yoga," "The Divine and Hostile Forces," page 382-389
7. The Mother, "The Mother's Agenda," 1962, Vol. 3, page 91
8. Ibid. page 101
9. Aurobindo, Sri, "Reason, Science and Yoga," page 222-224
10. Govindan, M. "Babaji and the 18 Siddha Kriya Yoga Tradition"
11. The Mother, "The Mother's Agenda," Vol. 3, Aug. 28, page 320-323
12. Chapple and Viraj, page 104-105
13. The Mother, "The Mother's Agenda," October 30, page 397-401

Chapter 4: KAIVALYA-PĀDA

1. Aurobindo, Sri, "Glossary of Terms in Sri Aurobindo's Writings," 1978, page 221
2. Aurobindo, Sri, "The Synthesis of Yoga" and "The Divine Life"
3. Feuerstein, G. "The Yoga Sūtras of Patañjali," page 142
4. Aurobindo, Sri, "The Divine Life"
5. Govindan, M. "Babaji and the 18 Siddha Kriya Yoga Tradition," page 126-133
6. Aurobindo, Sri, "Savitri"
7. The Mother, "The Mother's Agenda"
8. Aurobindo, Sri, "Sri Aurobindo on Himself," page 143-172
9. Purani, A.B. Evening Talks with Sri Aurobindo, 1959, page 45
10. The Mother, "The Mother's Agenda," vol. 3, 1962, Sept. 5, page 336
11. Hauer, J.W. "Der Yoga," 1958, page 283-284
12. Aurobindo, Sri, "Collected Works," Centennial Edition, volume XXIII, page 637
13. Chapple, Chris and Viraj, Yogi Anand (Eugene Kelly), "The Yoga Sutras of Patanjali," page 111

14. Rimpoche, Lati and Hopkins, Jeffrey, "Death, Intermediate State and Rebirth in Tibetan Buddhism," page 45
15. Feuerstein, G. "The Yoga Sūtras of Patañjali," page 142
16. *Shantideva.* "A Guide to the Bodhisattva Way of Life," 1992, page 193
17. Vyasa, *Vasitha, Book 5, chapter 77*
18. M. Govindan, "Babaji and the 18 Siddha Kriya Yoga Tradition," page 126-132
19. Ibid. page 135
20. Neelakantan, V.T., "Babaji's Masterkey to All Ills," 1953
21. P. Yogananda, "Autobiography of a Yogi," page 297-298

Bibliography

1. Translations

Aranya, Swami Hariharananda, "Yoga Philosophy of Patanjali," 1981, University of Calcutta Press, 48 Hazra Road, Calcutta, 700019

Chapple, Christopher and Yogi Anand Viraj (Eugene P. Kelly Jr.). The Yoga Sutras of Patanjali: An Analysis of the Sanskrit with Accompanying English Translation. Delhi: Sri Satguru Publications, 1990.

Elenjimittam, Anthony, The Yoga Philosophy of Patanjali, Allahabad: St. Paul Society, 1974.

Feuerstein, Georg, "Yoga-Sutra of Patanjali: A New Translation and Commentary," 1989, Inner Traditions, One Park Street, Rochester, Vermont 05767

Satchitananda, Swami, "The Yoga Sutras of Patanjali," 1978, Integral Yoga Publications, Yogaville, Route 1, Box 172, Buckingham, Virginia, 23921

2. Publications cited:

Aurobindo, Sri, "Letters on Yoga," Sri Aurobindo Ashram, Pondicherry, India, 605001; Available through Lotus Light Publications, Box 325, Twin Lakes, Wisconsin, 53181

Aurobindo, Sri, "Sri Aurobindo on Himself, Reminiscences and Observations," Available through Lotus Light Publications, Box 325, Twin Lakes, Wisconsin, 53181

Feuerstein, Georg, "Holy Madness: The Shock Tactics and Radical Teachings of Crazy Wise Adepts, Holy Fools and Rascal Gurus," 1991, Paragon House, 90 Fifth Ave, New York, N.Y. 10011

Ganapathy, T.N., "The Philosophy of the Tamil Siddhas," 1993, Indian Council of Philosophical Research. Distributed by Affiliated East West Press Pvt., Ltd. G-1/6 Ansari Road, Daryaganj, New Delhi, 110002, 1/1 General Patters Road, Madras 600002

Govindan, M. "Babaji and the 18 Siddha Kriya Yoga Tradition," 8th edition, 2005, Kriya Yoga Publications, 196 Mountain Road, P.O. Box 90, Eastman, Quebec, Canada, J0E 1P0

Govindan, M. Editor, "Thirumandiram: A Classic of Yoga and Tantra," by Siddhar Thirumoolar, 3rd printing, 2003, Kriya Yoga Publications, 196 Mountain Road, P.O. Box 90, Eastman, Quebec, Canada J0E 1P0

Hauer, J.W., "Der Yoga," Stuttgart, W. Kohlhammer Verlag, 1958

Kailasapathy, K. "The Writings of the Tamil Siddhas," The Saints: Studies in a Devotional Tradition of India.

Rose, Linda, "Your Mind: the Owner's Manual," 2nd edition, 2004, Kriya Yoga Publications, 196 Mountain Road, P.O. Box 90, Eastman, Quebec, Canada J0E 1P0

Shantideva. A Guide to the Bodhisattva Way of Life. Dharamsala, India: Library of Tibetan Works and Archives, 1992.

Swatmarama, Swami, "Hatha Yoga Pradipika," 1993, Bihar School of Yoga.

The Mother, "Agenda of the Mother," Institut de Recherches Evolutives, 32 Avenue de l'Observatoire, Paris, France. Available through Lotus Light Publications, Box 325, Twin Lakes, Wisconsin, USA, 53181

Venkatesananda, Swami, "The Concise Yoga Vasistha," 1984, State University of New York Press, University Plaza, Albany, New York, 12246

White, David Gordon, "The Alchemical Body: Siddha Traditions in Medieval India," 1996, University of Chicago, Press, Chicago, Illinois, 60637

Yogananda, Paramahansa, "The Autobiography of a Yogi," 1946, reprint 1996, Crystal Clarity Publishers, Nevada City, California, 95959

Zvelebil, Kamil V. "The Poets of the Powers: Freedom, Magic and Renewal," Integral Publishing, Lower Lake, California, 1993. Now solely distributed by Kriya Yoga Publications, St. Etienne de Bolton, Quebec, Canada, J0E 1P0

3. References

Apte, V.S. "The Practical Sanskrit-English Dictionary." Vols I-III. Poona: Prasad Prakashan, 1995.

Hiriyanna, M. "The Essentials of Indian Philosophy." Delhi: Motilal Banarsidass, 1995.

Monier-Williams, M. "A Sanskrit-English Dictionary." Delhi: Motilal Banrsidass, 1997.

Rimpoche, Lati, and Hopkins, Jeffrey. "Death, Intermediate State and Rebirth in Tibetan Buddhism." Ithaca, NY: Snow Lion, 1985.

Yocum, Glenn E. "Hymns to the Dancing Siva: A Study of Māṇikkavācakar's *Tiruvācakam.*" New Delhi: Heritage Publishers, 1982.

Index of Sanskrit Words in the Sūtras

(The following Sanskrit terms appear in their Sanskrit not English alphabetical order. See page xi "Guide to Pronunciation of Sanskrit" for the Sanskrit alphabetic order).

a

ā

i

ī

g

c

d

P

ph

b

bh

y

r

l

ś

s

h

Index of English words in the Sūtras Translation and Commentary

Index of Kriyas Indicated in the Yoga Sutras

About the Author Marshall Govindan

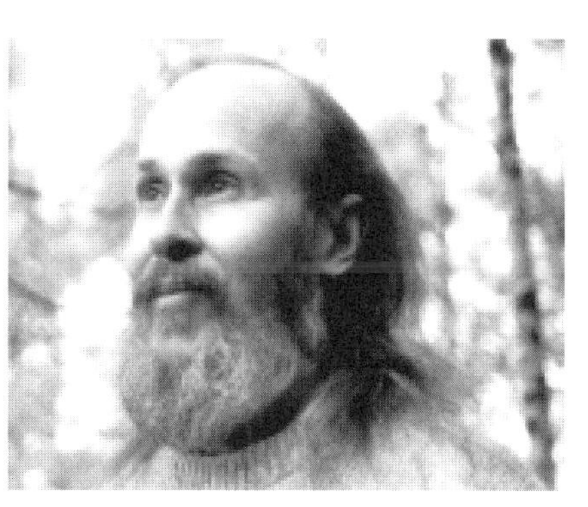

Marshall Govindan has practiced Babaji's Kriya Yoga intensively since 1969. He studied and practiced Kriya Yoga in India for five years with Yogi S.A.A. Ramaiah, assisting him in the establishment of 23 yoga centers around the world during an 18 year period. During this period he practiced Kriya Yoga for eight hours per day on average, and as a result attained Self-realization.

While in India he studied the Tamil language and the works of the Tamil Yoga Siddhas. In 1980 he assisted in the collection and publication of the complete writings of Siddhar Boganathar. In 1986 he administered the construction of a rehabilitation hospital dedicated to Yoga therapy and physical therapy in Tamil Nadu, India. In 1988 he was asked by Babaji Nagaraj, the founder of Kriya Yoga to begin teaching. In 1991, he wrote the best selling book, "Babaji and the 18 Siddha Kriya Yoga Tradition", now published in 13 languages. In 1992 he established Babaji's Kriya Yoga Ashram in St. Etienne de Bolton, Quebec. Classes, seminars and retreats are offered there year round.

In 1995 he retired from his work as the chief systems auditor for Quebec's largest employer, the cooperative Mouvement Desjardins to devote himself full time to teaching and publishing in the field of Yoga. Since then, he has travelled extensively throughout the world guiding about 50 Kriya Yoga study groups in over 20 countries, an ashram in Bangalore, India, and a lay order of teachers of Kriya Yoga: Babaji's Kriya Yoga Order of Acharyas, a non-profit educational charity, incorporated in the USA, Canada and India. Since 1989 he has personally initiated over 10, 000 persons in Babaji's Kriya Yoga in a series of intensive sessions and retreats.

In October 1999 he was blessed with the darshan of Babaji Nagaraj near his ashram in Badrinath, Himalayas.

He is currently co-directing a team of scholars in a large scale research project encompassing the whole of literature related to the Yoga of the Tamil Siddhas.

He is a graduate of Georgetown University School of Foreign Service and George Washington University in Washington, D.C.

Other titles available from Kriya Yoga Publications, Inc.:

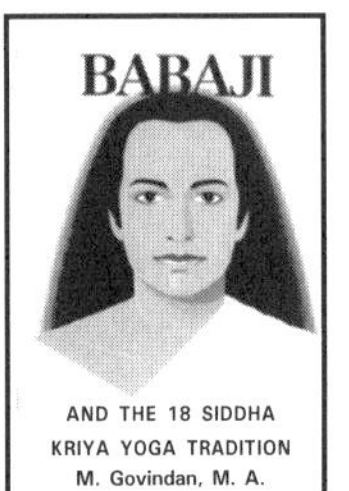

BABAJI and the 18 Siddha Kriya Yoga Tradition

new 8th edition

by M. Govindan

A rare account of Babaji, the Himalayan master who developed Kriya Yoga, the Siddhas, his source of inspiration and the principles of Kriya Yoga. Guidelines for its practice.216 pages, 4 maps, 33 color photos, 6" x 9".ISBN 1-895383-00-5. Canada: CN$30.76, U.S.A.: US$24.95, Asia & Europe: US$31.45

THIRUMANDIRAM:

A Classic of Yoga and Tantra

by Siddhar Thirumoolar

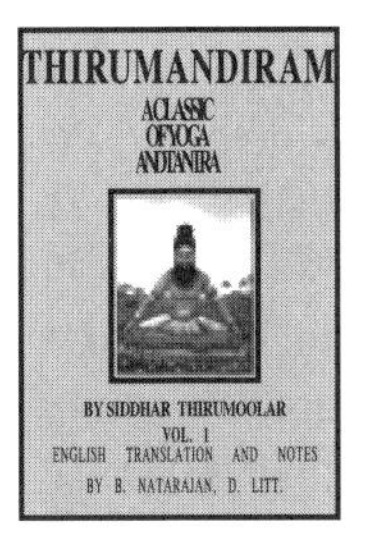

Edited by M. Govindan. Get connected to the roots of Yoga with the first English translation of Thirumoolar's classic masterpiece of Yoga, tantra, and Saiva Siddhantha, the gospel of the Tamil Yoga Siddhas. "The Thirumandiram is as important as the *Bhagavad Gita, The Sutras of Patanjali* and *Yoga Vasistha...*". This outstanding text is now available in a fine 3-volume edition, thanks to Marshall Govindan's labor of love" - Georg Feuerstein, Ph.D., contributing editor of *Yoga Journal.* 3,047 gem-like verses, with introduction, explanatory notes, index, glossary, illustrations. 828 pages in 3 volumes, 6" x 9". ISBN 1-895383-02-1. Canada: CN$58.32, U.S.A.: US$49.25, Asia & Europe: US$76.75

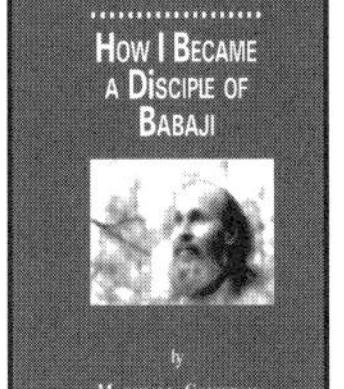

HOW I BECAME A DISCIPLE OF BABAJI

by M. Govindan

From early years of seeking through ascetic trials in India and Sri Lanka, filled with adventure and difficulties, the author shares a rare story with unusual candor and courage. His inspiring story provides rare insights into a little known world. 90 pages. 38 photographs, 6" x 9". ISBN 1-895383-04-8. Canada: CN$19.26, U.S.A.: US$12, Asia & Europe: US$14

BABAJI'S KRIYA HATHA YOGA: 18 Postures of Relaxation

by M. Govindan

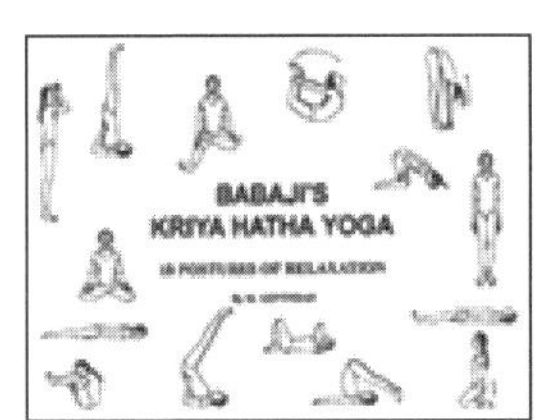

An efficient system developed by Babaji for rejuvenating the physical body, taught in stages and pairs with numerous benefits explained. ISBN 1-895383-03-X. 30 pages. 8 1/2" X 6 1/4". Canada: CN$11.77, USA: US$9.50, Asia & Europe: US$12

To order our publications or tapes:

Call toll free: 1-888-252-9642 or (450) 297-0258, Fax: (450) 297-3957, E-mail: info@babaji.ca

You may have your order charged to a VISA/MasterCard/Amex or send a cheque or International money order to: Kriya Yoga Publications, P.O. Box 90, Eastman, Quebec, Canada, J0E 1P0

All prices include shipping charges and taxes.

or place your order securely via our E-commerce at www.babaji.ca

THE YOGA OF SIDDHA BOGANATHAR

by T.N. Ganapathy, P.h.D

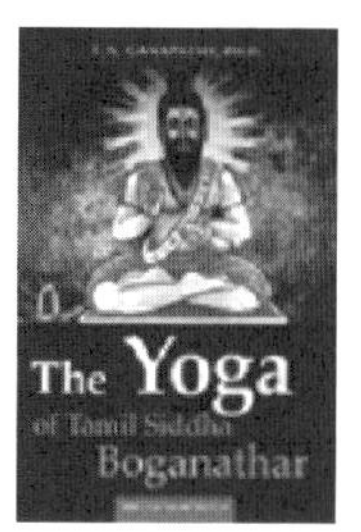

Boganathar was the guru of Kriya Babaji Nagaraj. Boganathar lived an extremely long life through the use of alchemy and special breathing techniques. He traveled all over the world and provided his disciples an illumined path to Self-realization and integral transformation of human nature into divinity. His astounding life provides a shining example of our human potential. The present work provides a biography of Boganathar, and **a translation and commentary of many of his poems.** ISBN 1-895383-19-6. **Vol. 1** Canada: CN$34.72, USA: US$24.95, Asia & Europe: US$31.45. **Vol. 2** Canada: CN$38.47, USA: US$33.45, Asia & Europe: US$60.95

THE VOICE OF BABAJI: A Trilogy on Kriya Yoga

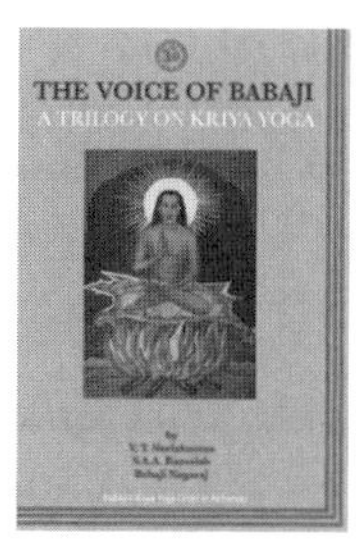

Sri V.T. Neelakantan recorded verbatim a series of talks given by Satguru Kriya Babaji in 1953. These are a fountain of delight and inspiration, illuminating the Kriya Yoga path towards God realization, unity in diversity and universal love. They also reveal the magnetic personality of Babaji and how he supports us all, with much humour and wisdom. 216 pages, 4 maps, Includes the fascinating accounts of the meetings with Babaji in Madras and in the Himalayas by authors V.T. Neelakantan and Yogi S.A.A. Ramaiah. Out of print for nearly 50 years, they are profound and important statements from one of the world's greatest living spiritual masters. 8 pages in color. 534 pages. ISBN 1-895383-23-4. Canada: CN$43.34, USA: US$34.50, Asia & Europe: US$48.50

THE YOGA OF THE 18 SIDDHAS: An Anthology

Edited by T.N. Ganapathy

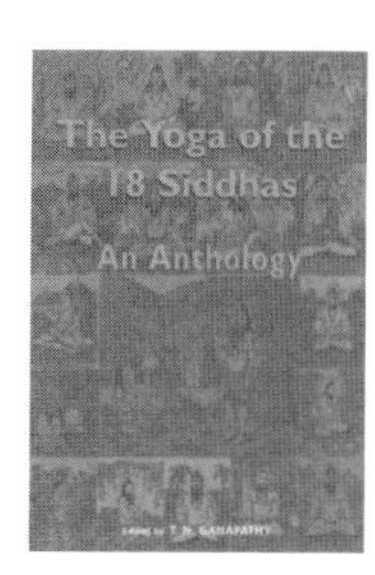

The Yoga of the Eighteen Siddhas: An Anthology includes a biography, an English translation and commentary of selected poems for each of the 18 Siddhas. It contains not only revolutionary statements of those great men and women who have reached the furthest heights of human potential, but also serves as a roadmap for the rest of us to follow. The Siddhas who represent the best of what we can all aspire to become have given us illuminated writings, so filled with the light of God realization that they can have an impact on our heart and mind, just by studying them. This book takes us along a path of Jnana Yoga. 642 pages. ISBN 1-895383-24-2. Canada: CN$49.22, USA: US$35.45, Asia & Europe: US$62.95

BABAJI'S KRIYA HATHA YOGA SELF-REALIZATION THROUGH ACTION WITH AWARENESS

DVD or VHS

With Marshall Govindan & Durga Ahlund

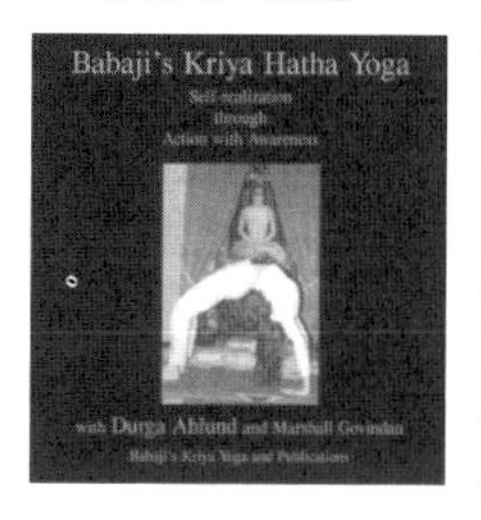

Learn the 18 postures developed by Babaji Nagaraj and become the Seer, not the Seen! Become aware of what is aware! Bliss arises! This unique, beautiful, 2 hour video provides careful detailed instructions in not only the technical performance of each posture, but also in the higher states of consciousness which they awaken. Make your practice of yoga deeply meditative. Taught in progressive stages with preparatory variations making them accessible to the beginner and challenging for the experienced student of Yoga. **"Earnest, unique and inspiring" - Yoga Journal.** ISBN 1-895383-18-8. Canada: CN$34.78, Quebec: CN$37.38, USA: US$28.45, Asia & Europe: US$31.95

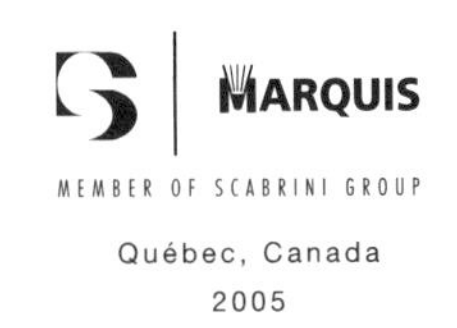

Québec, Canada
2005